SpringerBriefs in Food, Hea and Nutrition

MW00713594

Springer Briefs in Food, Health, and Nutrition present concise summaries of cutting edge research and practical applications across a wide range of topics related to the field of food science.

Editor-in-Chief
Richard W. Hartel
University of Wisconsin—Madison, USA

Associate Editors
J. Peter Clark, *Consultant to the Process Industries, USA*
David Rodriguez-Lazaro, *ITACyL, Spain*
David Topping, *CSIRO, Australia*

For further volumes:
http://www.springer.com/series/10203

Are Hugo Pripp

Statistics in Food Science and Nutrition

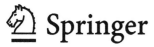 Springer

Are Hugo Pripp
Oslo University Hospital
Oslo, Norway

ISBN 978-1-4614-5009-2   ISBN 978-1-4614-5010-8 (eBook)
DOI 10.1007/978-1-4614-5010-8
Springer New York Heidelberg Dordrecht London

Library of Congress Control Number: 2012945941

Printed on acid-free paper

Springer is part of Springer Science+Business Media (www.springer.com)

Preface

A brief book will by its nature represent a compromise between methodological principles in statistics and epidemiology necessary to understand the subject and issues that are specific to the application of statistics to food science and nutrition. Therefore, the part on the methods and principles of statistics and epidemiology will cover these issues in a concise and basic manner. However, food scientists interested in statistics and epidemiology are urged to take general courses or read one of the many recommended textbooks in this area. The field of statistics is very large, and the number of journals and books is, fortunately, growing. For instance, www. springerlink.com lists 102 books available (as of April 2012) with the word *statistics* in its title.

Chapter 2, "Methods and Principles of Statistical Analysis," provides a concise introduction to the most important principles but with an edited reference to many of the excellent textbooks available. Readers who are unfamiliar with the basics of these principles are encouraged to consult more comprehensive textbooks or take courses in statistics, research methodology, and epidemiology.

The remaining chapters will be devoted to specific topics of interest in food science and nutrition. A primary goal of food producers is to make foods of excellent quality. Therefore, Chap. 3 concerns statistics in relation to product quality and sensory analysis. The relationship between food, lifestyle, and health is more important now than ever. The number of nutritional studies is quickly expanding, and their findings are discussed in the mass media. Health claims (or risks) are being reported to the public with increasing frequency, but are the claims based on rigorous research and proper statistical analysis? In this connection, Chap. 4 will focus on nutritional epidemiology and the health effects of foods. The topic of food and health is becoming ever more vital and closely linked to other lifestyle issues such as malnutrition or obesity, for example. Proper study design and statistical analysis are therefore of core importance. Chapter 5 – the last one in this Springer Brief – is titled the "Application of Multivariate Statistics: Benefits and Pitfalls." Food science and technology have been closely linked to the innovative use of novel multivariate statistics. These methods have been shown to have many applications and to confer numerous benefits in data analysis, and they are used especially in such areas as

spectroscopy, chemometrics, and sensory analysis. However, their complex statistical-mathematical nature is not without pitfalls. Pretreatment of data and subsequent
interpretation of results may be an issue. Thus, one should have a basic understanding of the methods' statistical principles before applying them extensively.

   With an educational and scientific background in food science and statistics, I
have had an ongoing personal interest in finding areas where the two topics inter-
twine. The many inspiring discussions on study design and statistical analysis with
medical researchers at Oslo University Hospital have also been instrumental to my
understanding of both the possibilities and limitations of statistics and, sometimes,
the beauty of a simple statistical test. I would like to thank Susan Safren and Rita
Beck at Springer New York for their continuous interest and patience in the prepara-
tion of this text. Special thanks go to my parents for always encouraging me.

Norway   Are Hugo Pripp

Contents

Chapter 1
Statistics in Food Science and Nutrition

Abstract Food and nutrition is not limited to cuisine, culture, and healthy living; it is also filled with the joy of data and statistics. Major innovations in statistics have come about from applied problems in food science. "The lady tasting tea" experiment and the relationship between Guinness and the t-test are classic examples. A fundamental knowledge of statistical analysis and study design is more important than ever, especially for investigating the relationship between food habits, health, and lifestyle.

Keywords William Sealy Gosset • Ronald A. Fisher • Food epidemiology

1.1 The Food Statistician

Perhaps you enjoy reading food labels on packages in the supermarket to know the content of protein, fat, and carbohydrates and other nutritional facts. Consumers are interested in sales statistics on different food groups and expiration dates. The subject of food and nutrition is not all about tradition, culture, healthy living, and cuisine. It is also filled with the joy of collecting and analyzing data from existing databases, interviewing consumers, or producing them yourself in the laboratory. Quantitative research involves the collection of relevant data and their analysis. Scientific reasoning, theory, and conclusions depend largely on the interpretation of data. Food science and nutrition is filled with the assessment of data from physical, microbial, chemical, sensory, and commercial analysis. In such an interdisciplinary area filled with quantitative data, statistics is at the heart of food and nutrition research.

From a very applied point of view, statistics can be divided into two subfields – descriptive statistics and statistical testing. Basic descriptive statistics are usually encountered long before one enters the field of professional food and nutrition

A.H. Pripp, *Statistics in Food Science and Nutrition*, SpringerBriefs in Food, Health, and Nutrition, DOI 10.1007/978-1-4614-5010-8_1,
© Springer Science+Business Media New York 2013

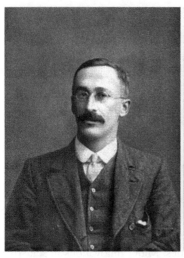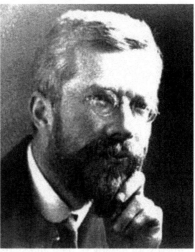

Fig. 1.1 William Sealy Gosset (*left*) (reproduced from Annals of Human Genetics, 1939: 1-9, with permission from John Wiley and Sons) and Ronald A. Fisher (*right*) are both regarded as being among the foremost founding fathers of modern statistics. Their methodological innovations in statistics were developed from agricultural and food scientific applications (see, e.g., Box 1978; Plackett and Bernard 1990)

research. The idioms "a picture is worth a thousand words" and "not seeing the forest for the trees" summarize what descriptive statistics is all about. It describes how descriptive statistics facilitates the interpretation of data and results. Typical examples are bar charts, trend lines, and scatter plots. Its application and usefulness is obvious also beyond the scientific (and statistical) community.

Statistical testing or inference, on the other hand, may not always be so intuitive, and its usefulness may be questioned outside the scientific community. It involves such expressions as significance, p-values, confidence intervals, and probability distributions and is founded on mathematics. One might have heard comments like "There are three kinds of lies: lies, damned lies, and statistics." The mathematics and accusations of aside, consider the following questions: Are your data due to a "real" effect or just a coincidence? Would you obtain the same results if you repeated the measurements, study, or experiment? What if the experiment were repeated and those data gave a different conclusion? If the results are due to coincidence or randomness, the results do not reflect a "real" effect. Statistical testing based on mathematical techniques say something about the probability that the outcome is not just a coincidence and about what the "real" effect is. Mathematics is the basic tool, but its application and interpretation depend on the scientific knowledge in your field of research. This is indeed the case as one moves from simple statistical tests to more complex statistical models known as analysis of variance, regression analysis, general linear model, logistic regression, and generalized linear models. These tests are actually quite related to each other, even though they have very different names.

1.2 Historical Anecdotes Relating Statistics to Food Science and Nutrition

What do drinking a pint of Guinness and a cup of tea with milk have in common? They have triggered fundamental innovations in statistical theory from applied problems in food science.

William Sealy Gosset, a chemistry graduate from Oxford, took up a job at Arthur Guinness, Son & Co, Ltd, in Dublin, Ireland. His task was to apply scientific methods to beer processing. To brew a perfect beer, exact amounts of yeast had to be mixed with the continuously fermenting barley. The amount of yeast was quantified by counting colonies. Gosset's challenge was to develop a method to quantify the amount of yeast colonies in entire jars of brewing beer based on small samples taken from the jars. This applied problem in food technology triggered an innovation in mathematics and statistics. He presented a report to the Guinness Board titled "The Application of the 'Law of Error' to the Work of the Brewery." Guinness Breweries did not allow its scientists to publish articles, but Gosset was granted permission provided he used a pseudonym and did not reveal any confidential data (Plackett and Bernard 1990; Raju 2005). Two papers were published in the statistical journal *Biometrika* under the pseudonym "Student" entitled "On the error of counting with a hemacytometer" (Student 1907) and "The probable error of a mean" (Student 1908). The last paper is a classic describing the test that became the well-known (Student's) *t*-test. Gosset continued to write statistical papers based on applied problems encountered in the brewery. Student's *t*-test and the t-distribution are used extensively in all types of applied statistics, but their applied origin is in food science and technology.

The "lady tasting tea" is the famous anecdote of an encounter with a woman by R.A. Fisher – one of the founding fathers of modern statistics and experimental design (Box 1978; Sturdivant 2000). His principles on statistical analysis and especially randomized designs are used in such experimental fields as agriculture, food science, and medicine. The title refers to the investigation of an English lady's claim that she could tell whether milk was poured into a cup first and then tea or first the tea and then milk. This is the account of what had a major impact on modern statistics according to Box (1978).

> Already, quite soon after he (i.e. R. A. Fisher) had come to Rothamstead, his presence had transformed one commonplace tea time to an historic event. It happened one afternoon when he drew a cup of tea from the urn and offered it to the lady beside him, Dr. B. Muriel Bristol, an algologist. She declined it, stating that she preferred a cup into which the milk had been poured first. "Nonsense," returned Fisher, smiling, "Surely it makes no difference." But she maintained, with emphasis, that of course it did. From just behind, a voice suggested, "Let's test her." It was William Roach who was not long afterward to marry Miss Bristol. Immediately, they embarked on the preliminaries of the experiment, Roach assisting with the cups and exulting that Miss Bristol divined correctly more than enough of those cups into which tea had been poured first to prove her case.

Regardless of whether or not the experiment was actually run, the statistical test developed to analyze a cross-table from this small sample of tea cups and the principles of randomly assigning samples of tea with milk poured first or after the tea are in common use. The mathematical-statistical test is called "Fisher's exact test," and the principle of randomization is fundamental in experimental studies and perhaps nowadays most closely linked to medical sciences and randomized clinical trials in drug development. However, its important origin is, again, linked to food science and technology.

R.A. Fisher's work on experimental data at the Rothamsted Experimental Station, located at Hertfordshire, England, on crop cultivation led to numerous innovations in modern statistics. He pioneered the principles of randomization and design of experiments and developed statistical methods such as analysis of variance and the foundation of maximum-likelihood estimations. Many of these innovations were presented in his 1925 book *Statistical Methods for Research Workers* and the later book *Design of Experiments*, published in 1935. Both books are regarded as reference texts in statistical science. Again, their applied origin that triggered important innovations in experimental and statistical science were rooted in agriculture and closely linked to food science and technology.

1.3   Why Statistics, Experimental Design, and Epidemiology Matter

Food scientists encounter many types of data. Consumers report their preferences, sensory panels give scores on selected scales, laboratories conduct chemical and microbial analyses, and companies set specific targets on production costs and sales. New ingredients may improve the technological properties in foodstuffs, but how should one conduct a study to test if it is worth changing the production process? How does one take into account other factors that might have an effect? How many samples should one test – 5, 10, 35, 178, or even more? Does it matter if data are collected from the same sample repeatedly over time compared to a "fresh" sample for each data point? All this is very important when it comes to describing data and experimental studies with an appropriate design and statistical methods.

Epidemiology is the study of the distribution and patterns of health events, health characteristics, and their causes or influences on well-defined populations. It is the cornerstone method of public health research and identifies risk factors for disease and targets for preventive medicine (see, e.g., Rothman et al. 2008). A balanced and appropriate diet has since ancient times been related to health and the prevention of disease. Food and nutritional epidemiology as a scientific discipline has attracted increased interest in recent years (Michels 2003). A large number of observational studies have attempted to elucidate the role of diet in health and disease. Since diet is strongly related to other aspects of life, because of the long exposure time and practical as well as ethical obstacles in assigning subjects to specific diets, randomized intervention studies are not as central in nutritional research as, for instance, in drug development. The effect of fats on the risk of coronary heart disease, the proportion of carbohydrates in one's diet and its effect on body mass index, and the onset of diabetes are all well-known examples of areas of concern in food epidemiology. A complicating issue is that individuals who try to eat a healthy diet are likely to lead a healthy lifestyle in general. This and other complex issues of food epidemiology can partly cause tabloid headlines about what type of food is "good" or "bad." It is therefore more important than ever to have a basic knowledge of epidemiological principles and of statistical methods to describe and analyze data from nutritional studies.

References

Box JF (1978) R. A. Fisher, the life of a scientist. Wiley, New York

Michels KB (2003) Nutritional epidemiology – past, present, future. Int J Epidemiol 32:486–488. doi:10.1093/ije/dyg216

Plackett RL, Bernard GA (1990) Student: a statistical biography of William Sealy Gosset. Clarendon, Oxford

Raju TNK (2005) William Sealy Gosset and William A. Silverman: two 'students' of science. Pediatrics 116:732–735. doi:10.1542/peds.2005-1134

Rothman KJ, Greenland S, Lash TL (2008) Modern epidemiology, 3rd edn. LWW, Philadelphia

Student JF (1907) On the error of counting with a haemacytometer. Biometrika 5:351–360

Student (1908) The probable error of a mean. Biometrika 6:1–25

Sturdivant R (2000) Lady tasting tea. Adapted from D Nolan and T Speed (2000) Mathematical statistics through applications. Springer, New York. http://www.dean.usma.edu/math/people/sturdivant/images/MA376/dater/ladytea.pdf. Accessed 1 Jun 2012

Chapter 2
Methods and Principles of Statistical Analysis

Abstract The best way to learn statistics is by taking courses and working with data. Some books may also be helpful. A first step in applied statistics is usually to describe and summarize data using estimates and descriptive plots. The principle behind p-values and statistical inference in general is covered with a schematic overview of statistical tests and models.

Keywords Recommended textbooks • Descriptive statistics • p-values • Statistical models

2.1 Recommended Textbooks on Statistics

How does one learn statistics, epidemiology, and experimental design? The recommended approach is, of course, to take (university) courses and combine it with applied use. In the same way it takes considerable effort and time to become trained in food technology or chemistry or as a physician, learning statistics – both the mathematical theory and applied use – takes time and effort. Some courses or books that promise to teach statistics without requiring much time and that neglect all the fundamental aspects of the subject could be deceiving. Learning the technical use of statistical software without some fundamental knowledge of what these methods express and the basics of calculations may leave the statistical analysis part in a black box. Appropriate statistical analysis and a robust experimental design should be the opposite of a black box – it should shed light upon data and give clear insights. It should ideally not be Harry Potter magic!

A comprehensive introduction to statistics and experimental design goes somewhat beyond the scope of this brief text. Therefore, this section will refer the reader to several excellent textbooks on the subject available from Springer. Readers with access to a university library service should be able to obtain these texts online through

A.H. Pripp, *Statistics in Food Science and Nutrition*, SpringerBriefs in Food, Health, and Nutrition, DOI 10.1007/978-1-4614-5010-8_2, © Springer Science+Business Media New York 2013

www.springerlink.com. Readers unfamiliar with the general aspects of statistics and experimental design or who have not taken introductory courses are encouraged to study some of these textbooks. An overview of the principles of descriptive statistics, statistical inference (e.g., estimations and p-values), classic tests, and statistical models is given later, but it is assumed that the reader has a basic knowledge of these principles.

2.1.1 Applied Statistics, Epidemiology, and Experimental Design

Statistics for Non-Statisticians by Madsen (2011) is an excellent introductory textbook for those new to the field. It covers the collection and presentation of data, basic statistical concepts, descriptive statistics, probability distributions (with an emphasis on the normal distribution), and statistical tests. The free spreadsheet software OpenOffice is used throughout the text. Additional material on statistical software, more comprehensive explanations on probability theory, and statistical methods and examples are provided in appendices and at the textbook's Web site. At 160 page, the textbook is not overwhelming. Readers with different interests, either in applied statistics or in mathematical-statistical concepts, are told which parts to read. Readers unfamiliar with statistics are highly encouraged to read this text or a similar introductory textbook on statistics.

Applied Statistics Using SPSS, STATISTICA, MATLAB and R by Marques de Sá (2007) is another recommended textbook, although it goes into somewhat more depth on mathematical-statistical principles. However, it provides a very useful introduction to using these four key statistical softwares for applied statistics. Combined with software manuals, it will give the reader an improved understanding of how to conduct descriptive statistics and tests. Both SPSS and STATISTICA have menu-based systems in addition to allowing users to write command lines (syntaxes). MATLAB and R might have a steeper learning curve and assume a more in-depth understanding of mathematical-statistical concepts, but they have many advanced functions and are used widely in statistical research. R is available for free and can be downloaded on the Internet. This is sometimes a great advantage and makes the user independent of updated licenses. Those who wish to make the effort to learn and use R will be part of a large statistical community (R Development Core Team 2012). It may, however, take some effort if one is unfamiliar with computer programming.

Biostatistics with R: An Introduction to Statistics Through Biological Data by Shahbaba (2012) gives a very useful step-by-step introduction to the R software platform using biological data. The many statistical methods available through so-called R packages and the (free) availability of the software makes it very attractive, but its somewhat more complicated structure compared to commercial software like SPSS, STATISTICA, or STATA might make it less relevant for those who use mostly so-called standard methods and have access to commercial software.

Various regression methods play a very important part in the analysis of biological data including food science and technology and nutrition research. *Regression Methods in Biostatistics* by Vittinghoff et al. (2012) gives an introduction to explorative and descriptive statistics and basic statistical methods. Linear, logistic, survival, and repeated measures models are covered without a too-overwhelming focus on mathematics and with applications to biological data. The software STATA that is widely used in biostatistics and epidemiology is used throughout the book.

Those who work much with nutrition, clinical trials, and epidemiology with respect to food will find very useful topics in textbooks such as *Statistics Applied to Clinical Trials* by Cleophas and Zwinderman (2012) and *A Pocket Guide to Epidemiology* by Kleinbaum et al. (2007). These books cover concepts that are statistical in nature but more related to clinical research and epidemiology. Clinical research is in many ways a scientific knowledge triangle comprised of medicine, biostatistics, and epidemiology.

Lehmann (2011) in his book *Fisher, Neyman, and the Creation of Classical Statistics* gives historical background of the scientists that laid the foundation for statistical analysis – Ronald A. Fisher, Karl Pearson, William Sealy Gosset, and Egon S. Pearson. Those with some insight into classical statistical methods and with a historic interest in the subject should derive much pleasure from reading about the discoveries that we sometimes take for granted in quantitative research. The text is not targeted at food applications but, without going into all the mathematics, provides a historical introduction to the development of statistics and experimental design. Some of the methods presented from their historical perspective might be difficult to follow if one is unfamiliar with statistics. However, a more comprehensive description of the "lady tasting tea" experiment is provided together with the many important concepts later discussed in relation to food science and technology.

2.1.2 Advanced Text on the Theoretical Foundation in Statistics

Numerous textbooks have a more theoretical approach to statistics, and many are collected in the series *Springer Texts in Statistics*. *Modern Mathematical Statistics with Applications* by Devore and Berk (2012) provides comprehensive coverage of the theoretical foundations of statistics. Another recommended text that gives an overview of the mathematics in a shorter format is the SpringerBrief *A Concise Guide to Statistics* by Kaltenbach (2011). These two and other textbooks with an emphasis on mathematical statistics are useful for exploring the fundamentals of statistical science with a more mathematical than applied approach to data analysis. However, most readers with a life science or biology-oriented background may find the formulas, notations, and equations challenging. Applied knowledge and mathematical knowledge often go hand in hand. It is usually more inspiring to learn the basic foundation if there is an applied motivation for a specific method. Many readers might therefore wish to consult textbooks with a more mathematical approach on "a-need-to-know" basis and begin with the previously recommended texts on applied use.

2.2   Describing Data

Food scientists encounter many types of data. Consumers report their preferences, sensory panels give scores on flavor and taste characteristics, laboratories provide chemical and microbial data, and management sets specific targets on production costs and expected sales. Analysis of all these data begins with a basic understanding of their statistical nature.

The first step in choosing an appropriate statistical method is to recognize the type of data. From a basic statistical point of view there are two main types of data – categorical and numerical. We will discuss them thoroughly before continuing with more specific types of data like ranks, percentages, and ratios. Many data sets contain missing data and extreme observations often called outliers. They also provide information and require attention.

To illustrate the different types of data and how to describe them, we will use yogurt as an example. Yogurt is a dairy product made from pasteurized and homogenized milk, fortified to increase dry matter, and fermented with the lactic acid bacteria *Streptococcus thermophilus* and *Lactobacillus delbrueckii subspecies bulgaricus*. The lactic acid bacteria ferment lactose into lactic acid, which lowers pH and makes the milk protein form a structural network, giving the typical texture of fresh fermented milk products. It is fermented at about 45°C for 5–7 h. A large proportion of yogurts also add fruit, jam, and flavor. There are two major yogurt processing technologies – stirring and setting. Stirred yogurt is fermented to a low pH and thicker texture in a vat and then pumped into packages, while set yogurt is pumped into packages right after lactic acid bacteria have been added to the milk; the development of a low pH and the formation of a gel-like texture take part in the package. The fat content can change from 0% fat to as high as 10% for some traditional types. It is a common nutritious food item throughout the world with a balanced content of milk proteins, dairy fats, and vitamins. In some yogurt products, especially the nonfat types, food thickeners are added to improve texture and mouthfeel (for a comprehensive coverage of yogurt technology see, e.g., Tamine and Robinson 2007).

2.2.1   Categorical Data

In Table 2.1 categorical and numerical data from ten yogurt samples are presented to illustrate types of data. The first three variables (flavor, added thickener, and fat content) are all derived from categorical data. Observations that can be grouped into categories are thus called categorical data. Statistically they contain less information than numerical data (to be covered later) but are often easier to interpret and

Table 2.1 Types of data and variables given by some yogurts samples

Type of data	Categorical			Numerical	
Type of variable	Nominal	Binary	Ordinal	Discrete	Continuous
Sample	Flavor	Added thickener	Fat content	Preference (1: low, 5: high)	pH
1	Plain	Yes	Fat free	1	4.41
2	Strawberry	Yes	Low fat	4	4.21
3	Blackberry	No	Medium	3	4.35
4	Vanilla	No	Full fat	4	
5	Vanilla	Yes	Full fat	4	4.15
6		No	Low fat	3	4.38
7	Strawberry	Yes	Fat free	2	4.22
8	Vanilla	Yes	Fat free	2	4.31
9	Plain	No	Medium	2	4.22
10	Strawberry	No	Full fat		6.41

understand. Low-fat yogurt conveys more clearly the fat content to most consumers than the exact fat content. Consumers like to know the fat content relative to other varieties and not the exact amount. Categorical data are statistically divided into three groups – nominal, binary, and ordinal data. Knowing the type of data one is dealing with is essential because that dictates the type of statistical analysis and tests one will perform.

Data that fall under nominal variables (e.g., "flavor" in Table 2.1) are comprised of categories, but there is no clear order or rank. Perhaps one person prefers strawberry over vanilla, but from a statistical point of view there is no obvious order to yogurt flavors. Other typical examples of numerical data in food science are food group (e.g., dairy, meat, vegetables), method of conservation (e.g., canned, dried, vacuum packed), and retail (e.g., supermarket, restaurant, fast-food chain). Statistically, nominal variables contain less information than ordinal or numerical variables. Thus, statistical methods developed for nominal variables can be used on other types of data, but with lower efficiency than other more appropriate or efficient methods.

If measurements can only be grouped into two mutually exclusive groups, then the data are called binary (also called dichotomous). In Table 2.1 the variable "added thickener" contains binary data. As long as the data can be grouped into only two categories, they should be treated statistically as binary data. Binary data can always be reported in the form of *yes* or *no*. Sometimes for binary data, *yes* and *no* are coded as 1 and 0, respectively. It is not necessary, but it is convenient in certain statistical analysis, especially when using statistical software. Binary variables are statistically often associated with giving the *risk* of something. One example is the risk of foodborne disease bacteria (also called pathogenic bacteria) in a yogurt sample. Pathogenic bacteria are either detected or not. However, from a statistical point of view the risk is estimated on a scale of 0 to 1, but for individual observations the risk is either present (pathogenic bacteria detected) or not (pathogenic bacteria not detected). Thus, it could then be presented as binary data for individual observations.

Data presented by their relative order of magnitude, such as the variable "fat content" in Table 2.1, are ordinal. Fat content expressed as fat free, low fat, medium fat, or full fat has a natural order. Since it has a natural order of magnitude with more than two categories, it contains more statistical information than nominal and binary data. Ordinal data can be simplified into binary data – e.g., reduced fat (combining the categories fat free, low fat, and medium fat) or nonreduced (full fat), but with a concomitant loss of information. Statistical methods used on nominal data can also be used on ordinal data, but again with a loss of statistical information and efficiency. If ordinal data can take only two categories, e.g., thick or thin, they should be considered binary.

2.2.2 Numerical Data

Observations that are measurable on a scale are numerical data. In Table 2.1, two types of numerical data are illustrated. These are discrete or continuous. In applied statistics both discrete and ordinal data are sometimes analyzed using methods developed for continuous data, even though it is not always appropriate according to statistical theory. Numerical data contain more statistical information than categorical data. Statistical methods suitable for categorical data analysis can therefore be applied to numerical data, but again with a loss of information. Therefore, it is common to apply other methods that take advantage of their additional statistical information compared with categorical data.

Participants in a sensory test may score samples on their preference using only integers like 1, 2, 3, 4, or 5. Observations that can take only integers (no decimals) are denoted discrete data. The "distance" between discrete variables is assumed to be the same. For instance the difference in preference between a score of 2 and 3 is assumed to be the same as the difference between scores 4 and 5. It is therefore possible to estimate, for example, the average and sum of discrete variables. If the "distance" cannot be assumed equal, discrete data should instead be treated as ordinal.

The pH of yogurt samples is an example of continuous data. Continuous data are measured on a scale and can be expressed with decimals. They contain more statistical information than the other types of data in Table 2.1. Thus, statistical methods applied to categorical or discrete data can be used on variables with continuous data, but not vice versa. For example, the continuous data on pH can be divided into those falling below and those falling above pH 4.6 and thereby be regarded as binary data and analyzed using methods for such data. However, if we have only information in our database about whether the yogurt sample is below or above pH 4.6, it is not possible to make such binary data continuous data. Thus, it is always useful to save the original continuous data even though they may be divided into categories for certain analysis. One may perhaps need the original data's additional statistical information at a later stage. Many advanced statistical methods like regression were first developed for continuous data as an outcome and then later expanded for use with categorical data.

2.2.3   Other Types of Data

Understanding the properties of categorical and numerical data serves as the foundation of quantitative and statistical analysis. However, in applied work with statistics one often encounters other specific types of data that require our attention. Some examples are missing data, ranks, ratios, and outliers. They have certain properties that one should be aware of.

Missing data are unobserved observations. Technical problems during laboratory analysis or participants' not answering all questions in a survey are typical reasons for missing data. In Table 2.1 yogurt samples 4, 6, and 10 have missing data for some of the variables. A main issue with missing data is whether there is an underlying reason why data are missing for some observations.

Statistical research on the effect of missing data is driven by medical statistics. It is a very important issue in both epidemiology and clinical studies and especially with longitudinal data (Song 2007; Ibrahim and Molenberghs 2009). What if a large proportion of those patients that do not experience any health improvement of a new drug drop out of a clinical trial? Statistical analysis could then be influenced greatly by the proportion of missing data and the biased medical conclusions that were reached. Missing data should therefore never be simply neglected or just replaced by a given value (e.g., the mean of nonmissing data) without further investigation. The issue of missing data is likewise important in food science and nutrition. We will use the terminology developed in medical statistics to understand how missing data could be approached.

Let us assume that we are conducting a survey on a new yogurt brand. We want to examine how fat content influences sensory preferences. A randomly selected group of 500 consumers is asked to complete a questionnaire about food consumption habits including their consumption of different yogurts. However, only 300 questionnaires are returned. Thus, we have 200 missing observations in our data set. According to statistical theory on missing data, these 200 missing observations can be classified as missing completely at random (MCAR), missing at random (MAR), or missing not at random (MNAR). This terminology is, unfortunately, not self-explanatory and somewhat confusing. However, one may say generally that it concerns the probability that an observation is missing.

Missing completely at random (MCAR): It is assumed here that the probability of missing data is unrelated to the possible value of a given missing observation (given that the observation was not missing and was actually made) or any other observations in one's data set. For instance, if the 200 missing observations were randomly lost, then it is unlikely that the probability to be missing is related to the preference scores of yogurt or any selected demographic data. Perhaps the box with the last 200 questionnaires was accidentally thrown away! For MCAR any piece of data is just as likely to be missing as any other piece of data. The nice feature is that the statistical estimates and resulting conclusions are not biased by the missing data. Fewer observations give increased uncertainty (i.e., reduced statistical power or consequently broader confidence intervals), but what we find is unbiased. They may just remain missing in your data set in further statistical analyses. All statistical analyses with MCAR give unbiased information on what influences yogurt preferences.

Missing at random (MAR): It is also assumed that the probability of missing data is unrelated to the possible value of a given missing observation (given that the observation was not missing and was actually made) but related to some other observed data in the data set. For example, if younger participants are less likely to complete the questionnaire than older ones, the overall analysis will be biased with more answers from older participants. However, separate analysis of young and old participants will be unbiased. A simple analysis to detect possible MAR in the data set entails examining the proportion of missing data between key baseline characteristics. Such characteristics in a survey could be the age, gender, and occupation of the participants.

Missing not at random (MNAR): Missing data known as MNAR present a more serious problem! It is assumed here that the probability of a missing observation is related to the possible value of a given missing observation (given that the observation was not missing and was actually made) or other unobserved or missing data. Thus, it is very difficult to say how missing data could influence one's statistical analysis. If participants who prefer low-fat yogurt are less likely to complete the questionnaire, then the results will be biased, but the information that it is due to their low preference for low-fat yogurt is lacking! The overall results will be biased and incorrect conclusions could be reached.

Whenever there are missing data, one needs to determine if there is a pattern in the missingness and try to explain why the data are missing. In Table 2.1 data on preference are missing for yogurt sample 10. However, the pH is exceptionally high. Perhaps something went wrong during the manufacture of the yogurt and the lactic acid bacteria did not ferment the lactose into lactic acid and so did not lower the pH. That could explain why preference was not examined for this sample. Therefore, always try to gather information to explain why data are missing. The best strategy is always to design a study in a way that minimizes the risk for missing data.

Especially in consumer surveys and sensory analysis, it is common to rank food samples. Ranking represents a relationship between a set of items such that, for any two items, the first is either ranked higher than, lower than, or equal to the second. For example, a consumer might be asked to rank five yogurt samples based on preference. This is an alternative to just giving a preference score for each sample. If there is no defined universal scale for the measurements, it is also feasible to use ranking for comparison of samples. Statistically speaking, data based on ranking have a lot in common with ordinal data, but they may be better analyzed using methods that take into account the ranks given by each consumer. It is therefore important to recognize rankings from other types of data.

A ratio is a relationship between two numbers of the same kind. We might estimate the ratio of calorie intake from dairy products compared with that from vegetables. Percentage is closely related as it is expressed as a fraction of 100. In Latin *per cent* means *per hundred*. Both ratios and percentages are sometimes treated as continuous data in statistical analysis, but this should be done with great caution. The statistical properties might be different around the extremes of 0 or 100%. Therefore, it is important to examine ratio and percentage data to assess how they should be treated statistically. Sometimes ratios and percentages are divided into ordinal categories if they cannot be properly analyzed with methods for continuous data.

Take a closer look at the data for sample 10 in Table 2.1. All the other samples have pH measurements around 4.5, but the pH of sample 10 is 6.41. It is numerically very distant from the other pH data. Thus, it might be statistically defined as an outlier, but it is not without scientific information. Since it deviates considerably from the other samples, the sample is likely not comparable with the other ones. This could be a sample without proper growth of the lactic acid bacteria that produce the acid to lower the pH during fermentation. Outliers need to be examined closely (just like missing data) and be treated with caution. With the unnatural high pH value of sample 10 compared with the other samples, the average pH of all ten samples would not be a good description of the typical pH value among the samples. Therefore, it might be excluded – or assessed separately – in further statistical analysis.

2.3 Summarizing Data

2.3.1 Contingency Tables (Cross Tabs) for Categorical Data

A contingency table is very useful for describing and comparing categorical variables. Table 2.2 is a contingency table with exemplified data to illustrate a comparison of preferences for low- or full-fat yogurt between men and women. The number of men and women in these data is different, so it is very useful to provide the percentage distribution in addition to the actual numbers. It makes the results much easier to read and interpret. Statistically, it does not matter which categorical variable is presented in rows or columns. However, it is rather common to have the variable defining the outcome of interest (preferred type of yogurt in our example) in columns and the explanation (gender of survey participants) in rows (Agresti 2002). In these illustrative data, women seem on average to prefer low-fat yogurt, and men seem to prefer full-fat yogurt. Perhaps this is a coincidence just for these 100 people, or is it a sign of a general difference in preference for yogurt types among men and women? Formal statistical tests and models are needed to evaluate this.

2.3.2 The Most Representative Value of Continuous Data

Let us examine again the pH measurements of our ten yogurt samples. Remember, we have missing data for sample 4; therefore, we have only nine data observations. Reordering the pH data in ascending yields 4.15, 4.21, 4.22, 4.22, 4.31, 4.35, 4.38,

Table 2.2 Comparison of two categorical variables

	Low-fat yogurt	Full-fat yogurt	Total
Men	12 (30%)	28 (70%)	40 (100%)
Women	45 (75%)	15 (25%)	60 (100%)
Total	60 (60%)	40 (40%)	100 (100%)

4.41, and 6.41. What single number represents the most typical value in this data set? For continuous data, the most "typical" value, or what is referred to in statistics as the central location, is usually given as either the mean or median. The mean is the sum of values divided by the number of values (the mean is also known as the "standard" average). It is defined for a given variable X with n observations as

$$\bar{x} = \frac{1}{n} \sum_{i=1}^{n} x_i$$

and is estimated in our example as

$$\text{mean} = \frac{4.15 + 4.21 + 4.22 + 4.22 + \mathbf{4.31} + 4.35 + 4.38 + 4.41 + 6.41}{9} = 4.52.$$

The single outlier measurement of pH 6.41 has a relatively large influence on the estimated mean. An alternative to the mean could be to use the median. The median is the numeric values separating the upper half of the sample or, in other words, the value in the middle of our data set. The median is found by ranking all the observations from lowest to highest value and then picking the middle one. If there is an even number of observations and thus no single middle value, then the median is defined as the mean of the two middle values. In our example the middle value is 4.31 (indicated by bold typeface in the equation estimating the mean). A rather informal approach to deciding whether to use the mean or median for continuous data is to estimate them both. If the median is close to the mean, then one can usually use the mean, but if they are substantially different, then the median is usually the better choice.

2.3.3   Spread and Variation of Continuous Data

Describing the central location or the most typical value is telling only half the story. One also needs to describe the spread or variation in the data. For continuous data it is common to use the standard deviation or simply the maximum and minimum values. These might not be so intuitive as the mean and median. If the data set has no extreme outliers or a so-called skewed distribution (many very high or low values compared with the rest of the data), it is common to use the standard deviation. It can be estimated for a given variable X with n observations as

$$\text{Standard deviation (SD)} = \sqrt{\dfrac{\sum_{i=1}^{n}(x_i - \bar{x})^2}{n-1}}$$

If we exclude the extreme pH value in sample 10 (regarded as an outlier), then the new mean of our remaining eight data points on pH is estimated to be 4.28 and the standard deviation is estimated as

$$\text{SD} = \sqrt{\dfrac{(4.41-4.28)^2 + (4.21-4.28)^2 + \ldots + (4.22-4.28)^2}{8-1}} = 0.09$$

Fortunately, most spreadsheets such as Excel or OpenOffice or statistical software can estimate standard deviations and other statistics efficiently and lessen the need to know the exact estimation formulas and computing techniques. If we assume that our data are more or less normally distributed, then a distance of one standard deviation from the mean will contain approximately 65% of our data. Two standard deviations from the mean will contain approximately 95% of our data. This is the main reason why continuous data are often described using the mean and standard deviation.

If a data set has a skewed distribution or contains many outliers or extreme values, it is more common to describe the data as the median, with the spread represented by the minimum and maximum values. To reduce the effect of extreme values, the so-called interquartile range is an alternative measure of spread in data. It is equal to the difference between the third and first quartiles. It can be found by ranking all the observations in ascending order. For the sake of simplicity, let us assume one has 100 observations. The lower boundary of the interquartile range is at the border of the first 25% of observations – in this example observation 25 if they are ranked in ascending order. The higher boundary of the interquartile range is at the border of the first 75% of observations – in this example observation 75 if they are ranked in ascending order.

2.4 Descriptive Plots

The adage "a picture is worth a thousand words" refers to the idea that a complex idea can be conveyed with just a single still image. Actually, some attribute this quote to the Emperor Napoleon Bonaparte, who allegedly said, "Un bon croquis vaut mieux qu'un long discours" (a good sketch is better than a long speech). We might venture to rephrase Napoleon to describe data – "A good plot is worth more

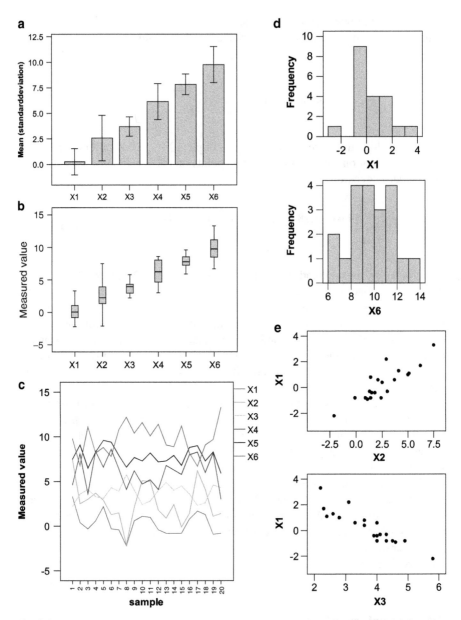

Fig. 2.1 Typically used descriptive plots. The plots are (**a**) bar chart, (**b**) box plot, (**c**) line plot, (**d**) histogram, and (**e**) scatterplot. All plots were made using data in Box 5.1 in Chap. 5

than a thousand data." Plots are very useful for describing the properties of data. It is recommended that these be explored before further formal statistical analysis is conducted. Some examples of descriptive plots are given in Fig. 2.1

2.4.1   Bar Chart

A bar chart or bar graph is a chart with rectangular bars with lengths proportional to the values they represent. They can be plotted vertically or horizontally. For categorical data the length of the bar is usually the number of observations or the percentage distribution, and for discrete or continuous data the length of the bar is usually the mean or median with (error) lines sometimes representing the variation expressed as, for example, the standard deviation or minimum and maximum values. Bar charts are very useful for presenting data in a comprehensible way to a nonstatistical audience. Bar charts are therefore often used in the mass media to describe data.

2.4.2   Histograms

Sometimes it is useful to know more about the exact spread and distribution of a data set. Are there many outliers, or is the data distribution equally spread out? To know more about this, one could make a histogram, which is a simple graphical way of presenting a complete set of observation in which the number (or percentage frequency) of observations is plotted for intervals of values.

2.4.3   Box Plots

A box plot (also known as a box-and-whisker diagram) is a very efficient way of describing numerical data. It is often used in applied statistical analysis but is not as intuitive for nonstatistical readers. The plot is based on a five-number summary of a data set: the smallest observation (minimum), the lower quartile (cutoff value of the lowest 25% of observations if ranked in ascending order), the median, the upper quartile (cutoff value of the first 75% of observations if ranked in ascending order), and the highest observation (maximum). Often the "whiskers" may indicate the 2.5% and 97.5% values with outliers and extreme values indicated by individual dots. Box plots provide more information about the distribution than bar charts. If the line indicating the median is not in the middle of the box, then this is usually a sign of a skewed distribution.

2.4.4   Scatterplots

Scatterplots are very useful for displaying the relationship between two numerical variables. These plots are also sometimes called XY-scatter or XY-plots in certain software. A scatterplot is a simple graph in which the values of one variable are plotted against those of the other. These plots are often the first step in the statistical analysis of the correlation between variables and subsequent regression analysis.

2.4.5   Line Plots

A line plot or graph displays information as a series of data points connected by lines. Depending on what is to be illustrated, the data points can be single observations or statistical estimates as, for example the mean, median, or sum. As with the bar chart, vertical lines representing data variation, for example standard deviation, may then be used. Line plots are often used if one is dealing with repeated measurements over a given time span.

2.5   Statistical Inference (the *p*-Value Stuff)

Descriptive statistics are used to present and summarize findings. This may form the basis for decision making and conclusions in, for example, scientific and academic reports, recommendations to governmental agencies, or advice for industrial production and food development. However, what if the findings were just due to a coincidence? If the experiment were repeated and new data collected, a different conclusion might be reached. With statistical methods it is necessary to assess whether findings are due to randomness and coincidence or are representative of the "true" or underlying effect. One set of tools is called statistical tests (or inference) and form the basis of *p*-values and confidence intervals.

The basis is a hypothesis that could be rejected in relation to an alternative hypothesis given certain conditions. In statistical sciences these hypotheses are known as the null hypothesis (typically a conservative hypothesis of no "real" difference between samples, no correlation, etc.) and the alternative hypothesis (i.e., that the null hypothesis is not "in reality" true). The principle is to assume that the null hypothesis is true. Methods based on mathematical statistics have been developed to estimate the probability of outcomes that are at least as "rare" as the observed outcomes, given the assumption that the null hypothesis is true. This probability is the well-known *p*-value. If this probability is small (typical less than 5%), then the null hypothesis is typically rejected in favor of the alternative hypothesis. The level of this probability before the null hypothesis is rejected is called the significance level (often denoted α).

The relationship between the (unknown) reality if the null hypothesis is true or not and the decision to accept or reject the null hypothesis is shown in Table 2.3. Two types of error can be made – Type I and Type II errors. The significance level – α – is typically set low (e.g., 5%) to avoid Type I errors that from a methodological point of view are regarded as being more "serious" than Type II errors. The null hypothesis is usually very conservative and assumes, for example, no difference between groups or no correlation. The Type II error is denoted by β. The statistical

Table 2.3 Two types of statistical errors: Types I and II errors and their relationship to significance level α and the statistical power $(1-\beta)$

	Null hypothesis (H_0) is true	Alternative hypothesis (H_1) is true
Accept null hypothesis	Correct decision	Type II error: β
Reject null hypothesis	Type I error: α	Correct decision

power is the ability of a test to detect a true effect, i.e., reject the null hypothesis if the alternative hypothesis is true. Thus, this is the opposite of a Type II error and consequently equal to $1-\beta$.

2.6 Overview of Classical Statistical Tests

Classical statistical tests are pervasive in research literature. More complex and general statistical models can often express the same information as these tests. Table 2.4 presents a list of some common statistical tests. It goes beyond the scope of this brief text to explain the statistical and mathematical foundations of these tests, but they are covered in several of the recommended textbooks. Modern software often has menu-based dialogs to help one determine the correct test. However, a basic understanding of their properties is still important.

2.7 Overview of Statistical Models

Generally speaking, so-called linear statistical models state that your outcome of interest (or a mathematical transformation of it) can be predicted by a linear combination of explanatory variables, each of which is multiplied by a parameter (sometimes called a coefficient and often denoted β). To avoid having the outcome be estimated as zero if all explanatory variables are zero, a constant intercept (often denoted β_0) is included. The outcome variable of interest is often called the dependent variable, while the explanatory variables that can predict the outcome are called independent variables.

The terminology in statistics and experimental design may sometimes be somewhat confusing. In all practical applications, models like linear regression, analysis of covariance (ANCOVA), analysis of variance (ANOVA), or general linear models (GLM) are very similar. Their different terminology is due as much to the historical tradition in statistical science as to differences in methodology. Many of these models with their different names and terminologies can be expressed within the framework of generalized linear models. It was common to develop mathematical methods to estimate parameter values and p-values that could be calculated manually by hand and

Table 2.4 Proposed statistical tests or models depending on properties of the outcome and explanatory variable. Nonparametric alternative is given in *brackets* if assumptions on normal distributions are not valid. The number of mentioned tests is limited and recommendations may vary depending on the nature of the data and purpose of analysis

Purpose with statistical analysis	Type of outcome data				
	Nominal	Binary	Ordinal	Discrete	Continuous
Against specific null hypothesis about expected mean or proportion	Chi-squared test	Binomial test	Chi-squared test	One sample t-test	One sample t-test
Relationship with continuous explanatory variable	"Use a statistical model"	"Use a statistical model"	Spearman correlation	Pearson (Spearman) correlation	Pearson (Spearman) correlation
Difference in expected mean or proportions between two groups	Chi-squared test for cross tabs	Chi-squared test for crosstabs	Chi-squared test for crosstabs	Two-sample t-test (Mann–Whitney U test)	Two-sample t-test (Mann–Whitney U test)
Difference between mean or proportions between more than two groups	Chi-squared test for crosstabs	Chi-squared test for crosstabs	Chi-squared test for crosstabs	Analysis of variance (Kruskal–Wallis H test)	Analysis of variance (Kruskal–Wallis H test)
Analyzed as linear statistical model	Multinomial logistic regression	Binary logistic regression	Ordinal logistic regression	Linear regression/general linear model	Linear regression/general linear model
Two clustered or repeated measurements	McNemar–Bowker test	McNemar test	McNemar–Bowker test	Paired sample t-test (Wilcoxon signed-rank test)	Paired sample t-test (Wilcoxon signed-rank test)
Statistical model for clustered or repeated measurements	Mixed multinomial logistic regression or GEE	Mixed binary logistic regression or GEE	Mixed ordinal logistic regression or GEE	Linear mixed model or GEE	Linear mixed model or GEE

GEE generalized estimating equations

with the help of statistical tables. Most graduates in statistics are familiar with such methods for simple regression and ANOVA methods. However, recent innovations in mathematical statistics, and not least computers and software, have in an applied sense replaced such "manual" methods. These computer-assisted methods are usually based on the theory of so-called likelihood functions and involve finding their maximum values by using iterations. In other words, these are methods where computer software is needed for most applied circumstances. The theory behind maximum-likelihood estimations is covered in several of the more advanced recommended textbooks.

Linear statistical models are often described within the framework of generalized linear models. The type of model is determined by the properties of the outcome variable. A dependent variable with continuous data is usually expressed with an identity link and is often referred to by more traditional terms such as linear regression or analysis of variance. If the dependent variable is binary, then it is usually expressed by a logit link and is often referred to by the more traditional term logistic regression. Count data use a log link and the statistical model is traditionally referred to as Poisson regression (e.g., Dobsen and Barnett 2008).

References

Agresti A (2002) Categorical data analysis, 2nd edn. Wiley, Hoboken

Cleophas TJ, Zwinderman AH (2012) Statistics applied to clinical studies, 5th edn. Springer, Dordrecht

Devore JL, Kenneth N (2012) Modern mathematical statistics with applications, 2nd edn. Springer, New York

Dobsen AJ, Barnett A (2008) An introduction to generalized linear models, 3rd edn. CRC Press, London

Ibrahim JG, Molenberghs G (2009) Missing data methods in longitudinal studies: a review. Test 18:1–43. doi:10.1007/s11749-009–0138-x

Kaltenbach HM (2011) A concise guide to statistics. Springer, New York

Kleinbaum DG, Sullivan K, Barker N (2007) A pocket guide to epidemiology. Springer, New York

Lehmann EL (2011) Fisher, Neyman, and the creation of classical statistics. Springer, New York

Madsen B (2011) Statistics for non-statisticians. Springer, Heidelberg

Marques de Sá JP (2007) Applied statistics using SPSS, STATISTICA, MATLAB and R, 2nd edn. Springer, Berlin

Shahbaba R (2012) Biostatistics with R: an introduction to statistics through biological data. Springer, New York

Song PXK (2007) Missing data in longitudinal studies. In: Correlated data analysis: modeling, analytics, and applications. Springer, New York

Tamine AY, Robinson RK (2007) Tamine and Robinson's yoghurt science and technology, 3rd edn. CRC Press, Cambridge

R Development Core Team (2012) The R project for statistical computing. http://www.r-project.org. Accessed 30 Apr 2012

Vittinghoff E, Glidden DV, Shiboski SC, McCulloch CE (2012) Regression methods in biostatistics: linear, logistic, survival and repeated measures models, 2nd edn. Springer, New York

Chapter 3
Applying Statistics to Food Quality

Abstract To apply statistics to food quality, quality must be quantified, measured, and assessed. Statistical process control is the application of statistical methods to the monitoring and control of a process to ensure that it operates to produce conforming products. Control charts are used extensively. The term Six Sigma has its roots in statistical theory and the spread of data. Statistical methods are also fundamental to the assessment of results from sensory analysis. Shelf life and product quality can use many of the statistical methods from time-to-event analysis developed in medical statistics.

Keywords Food quality • Statistical process control • Six Sigma • Survival analysis

3.1 The Concept of Food Quality

What is food quality and how can it be measured and assessed? According to Wikipedia (2012), it is "The quality characteristics of food that is acceptable to consumers. This includes external factors as appearance (size, shape, colour, gloss, and consistency), texture, and flavour; factors such as federal grade standards (e.g. of eggs) and internal (chemical, physical, microbial)." The American Society for Quality defines quality as "a subjective term for which each person or sector has its own definition. In technical usage, quality can have two meanings: (1) the characteristics of a product or service that bear on its ability to satisfy stated or implied needs; (2) a product or service free of deficiencies. According to Joseph Juran, quality means 'fitness for use'; according to Philip Crosby, it means 'conformance to requirements'" (American Society for Quality 2012). Many food consumers also rely on manufacturing and processing standards, particularly in order to know what ingredients are present, due to dietary or nutritional requirements or medical conditions to assess quality. Food scientists focus on methods for monitoring food and nutritional quality, shelf life testing and validation, environmental factors affecting food quality, impact of present and proposed regulation, and statistical interpretation

A.H. Pripp, *Statistics in Food Science and Nutrition*, SpringerBriefs in Food, Health, and Nutrition, DOI 10.1007/978-1-4614-5010-8_3,
© Springer Science+Business Media New York 2013

of attributes expressing quality. The wide use of quality as a property and concept makes it challenging in food research with a statistical approach. Quality seems impossible to measure with one universal variable.

Food product quality has been defined in a variety of different ways (Lawless 1995; Lawless and Heymann 2010). For instance, sensory science – which is perhaps the subdiscipline within food science and technology closest to consumer preferences, perceptions, and the common understanding of quality – focuses on issues of consumer satisfaction as a measure of quality. Expert judges, commodity graders, or government inspectors who assess product quality also commonly use sensory analyses. This tradition is strongly related to the detection of well-known defects or expected problem areas.

Another strong tradition within the field of food quality is the emphasis on conformance to specifications. It is useful in manufacturing where certain attributes, properties, or performance can be measured using instrumental or objective means. Methods for statistical process control have made substantial contributions in this aspect of quality to reduce production variability (see, e.g., Oakland 2007).

Food quality is also related to fitness of use. It recognizes that quality does not exist as an isolated entity but is closely related to consumer preferences. Finally, the reliability or consistency in the sensory experience and performance of a food product has also been recognized as an important feature of product quality. Consumer expectations arise out of experience, and maintaining that experience goes a long way toward building consumer confidence and, thereby, a part of food quality.

3.2   Measuring Quality Quantitatively

Lawless (1995) raises the issue in his essay "Dimensions of sensory quality: A critique" of whether overall (food) quality can be measured. He concludes that it can, but only with great difficulty. Quality is bound to consumer perceptions, opinions, and attitudes. Individual aspects of quality can be quantified and optimized, but even this will not guarantee product success.

However, in the statistical analysis of quantitative research we rely on measurements and data to perform our evaluation. Even an ambiguous expression such as quality must be quantified. Food science and technology might find additional inspiration in quantifying aspects of quality from research in psychiatry, psychology, and behavioral sciences. Validated rating scales and questionnaires with equivalent clinical interpretations across study groups are developed for aspects – with somewhat ambiguous interpretations – such as physical disability, social health and psychological well-being, anxiety, depression, mental status testing, pain, general health status, and quality of life, among others (McDowell 2006). It is important to develop generally accepted rating scales for aspects of food quality that can be used across study groups and food commodities.

Quantitative research and statistical analysis are especially important in three aspects in producing foods with quality: statistical process control, statistical assessment of sensory data, and statistical assessment of shelf life. Most of the discussion here will focus on univariate approaches (statistical methods with only one outcome variable in the model). Multivariate statistical methods as principal component analysis will be briefly discussed, but a more thorough discussion on multivariate statistical analysis with its benefits and pitfalls will be covered in Chap. 5.

3.3 Statistical Process Control

3.3.1 The Foundation of Statistical Process Control

Statistical process control (SPC) was developed in the early 1920s by scientific pioneers like Walter A. Shewhart (1891–1967) and later developed to improve manufacturing quality during World War II. The method is very closely linked to the development of Japanese industry after the war and played a key role in their manufacture of products, that were often superior to their American or European counterparts. American scientists such as William Edwards Deming (1900–1993) were instrumental in introducing SPC to Japanese industry. SPC is the application of statistical methods to the monitoring and control of a process to ensure that it operates at its full potential to produce conforming product (Deming 1982). A fundamental goal of a process using SPC is to predictably produce as much conforming product as possible with the least possible waste. Ideally, it is a technique to prevent error rather than to detect it. Products of the required quality will be produced, not because they are inspected, but rather because they are manufactured properly.

Much of the power of SPC lies in the fact that it makes it possible to examine a process and the sources of variation in that process. The purpose of SPC is to find as many sources of variation as possible and then eliminate them (Bergman and Klefsjö 1994). This is based on objective analysis using statistical principles instead of subjective opinions. Quality characteristics must therefore be determined numerically. Variations in the process that may affect the quality of the end product or service can be detected and corrected, thereby reducing waste as well as the likelihood that problems will be passed on to the customer. With its emphasis on early detection and prevention of problems, SPC has a distinct advantage over other quality methods, such as inspection, that apply resources to detect and correct problems after they have occurred.

From a statistical point of view, SPC is linked to the logical phenomenon that there are variations in processes and, consequently, product characteristics. Statisticians, including those that work in the field of food science and nutrition, base their scientific reasoning (and daily income) on the fact that there exist natural inherent variations in observations of a process. Thus, an important principle in process quality control is to reduce variation to make sure that the output continues to meet the expected requirements. Therefore, a fundamental aspect of SPC is to identify the cause of variation from descriptive statistical analysis based on, for example, control charts. Typical sources of systematic variation in the food industry can be raw materials, wear of process machinery, or operator skills.

Fundamental to the efficient application of SPC is a thorough understanding of the production process and causes of variation in output to eliminate or reduce sources of specific variations. Application of statistical principles therefore represents an approach that differs from the traditional concept of inspection of each individual product for quality control. Key elements in SPC include the use of tools like control charts, a focus on continuous improvement, and designed experiments.

3.3.2   Control Charts

Control charts are graphical tools for monitoring a manufacturing process (Naikan 2008). Typically, a numerical value expressing a quality characteristic is plotted on the Y-axis against the sample number on the X-axis. Other diagrams that are commonly used in SPC include histograms, scatterplots, stem and leaf plots, and box plots, but the focus here will be on control charts since they are statistically very specific to SPC.

An important assumption underlying the use of control charts (and the application of SPC in general) is that the process variability is both known (or can be determined) and stable. Thus, the process can be said to be under statistical control. A typical control chart is shown in Fig. 3.1. Each point represents a statistic (e.g., mean, range, or proportion) of a measured quality characteristic in samples taken from the process at different times. A centerline represents the average value of the quality characteristics and indicates the center (or statistical mean) of the process. The upper action limit and the lower action limit are used to control the process. They are sometimes called natural process limits and are typically three standard errors from the centerline. The process is said to be in statistical control if all sample points plot inside these limits. For a process to be in control, the control chart should have no trends or nonrandom patterns. Optionally, a chart may also have lines indicating upper and lower warning limits. These are typically two standard errors above and below the centerline. Action and warning limits to control a process are not without their drawbacks and require a careful interpretation and understanding. It is quite possible, through the process of sampling and inherent variability, that there will be values outside the limits (outliers), even though no change has occurred in the underlying process. On the other hand, there may also be values within the control limits despite real changes in the process (Love 2007). The choice and application of the control limits represent a compromise between these two scenarios and can therefore be seen statistically related to Type I and Type II errors, the significance level and statistical power.

Three different types of control charts are especially relevant in SPC: average control charts, moving average control charts, and spread control charts.

Average control charts are very useful when group sizes are very large and changes occur slowly. A given number of n measurements give a group. The mean μ, standard deviation σ, and standard error of the mean σ_{SE} based on these n measurements can then be estimated. If the outcome is a continuous variable x in a group of n observations that is approximately normally distributed, then these can be estimated using the following equations:

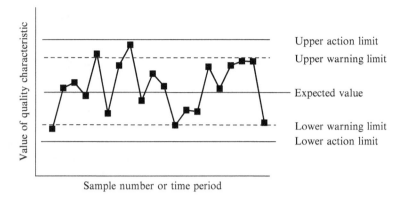

Fig. 3.1   Typical outline of a control chart used in statistical process control

$$\hat{\mu} = \overline{x} = \frac{1}{n}\sum_{i=1}^{n} x_i,$$

$$\hat{\sigma} = s = \sqrt{\frac{\sum_{i=1}^{n}(x_i - \overline{x})^2}{n-1}},$$

$$\hat{\sigma}_{SE} = \frac{\hat{\sigma}}{\sqrt{n}}.$$

The standard error of the mean can, according to statistical theory, be interpreted as the standard deviation of the estimated means. Thus, if the mean can be said to behave according to the central limit theorem, the mean ± 2 standard errors or ± 3 standard errors should contain, respectively, approximately 95% or 99% of all estimated means if the process is under statistical control.

An average control chart with upper and lower action limits and upper and lower warning limits is shown in Fig. 3.1. Interpretation of the control chart in SPC is based on simple rules (Love 2007). If any of the following rules apply, it may be taken as evidence that there is a change in the variability of the data and that some underlying cause must be present.

- One point lies outside either action limit.
- Two successive points lie outside the same warning limits.
- Seven successive points lie on one side of the mean.
- Seven successive points consistently either increase or decrease.

These rules may be less strict, but then they carry a greater probability of a statistical Type I error, i.e., false alarm – rejecting the null hypothesis of no change in the variability of the data when this null hypothesis is actually true!

Moving average control charts are most useful when the group sizes are small and changes occur quickly. At each sampling, evaluate the mean of the group of the last *m* values. The oldest observation is then discarded, the newest is included, and the average moves on. The moving average control chart is constructed and interpreted as described previously for average control charts.

Spread control charts estimate the mean spread of data. The spread of a group is the difference between the largest and smallest of the *m* values within that group. The mean spread is the average of the spread for all *n* groups.

3.3.3   The Statistics of Six Sigma

Six Sigma is a business management strategy, originally developed by Motorola, USA and is now used in many sectors of industry (Tennant 2001). Examples of large food companies that have adopted the Six Sigma strategy are Heinz, PepsiCo, and United Biscuits. The basic principle is again to improve the quality of processes by indentifying and removing the causes of defects (errors) and minimizing variability. Statistical methods and statistical process control are here an important tool. The term Six Sigma process comes from the notion that if one has six standard deviations between the process mean and the nearest specification limit, as illustrated in Fig. 3.2, then practically no items will fail to meet specifications. This is founded statistically on the so-called central limit theorem, which shows that if we plot the sample average of a process parameter, then it will tend to have a normal distribution. The normal distribution is described by its parameters mean (μ) and standard deviations (σ). For a normal distribution it can be shown that 99.7% of all points will fall within the 3σ limits on either side of the mean. If the distance to the specification limits are increased to 6σ, statistically as low as 0.0000002% will fall outside these limits. The upper and lower control limits of the control chart are thereby determined based on this principle. This means that almost all the data points will fall within 3σ control limits if the process is free from assignable causes. Even if the mean move right of left by 1.5σ, the process is within good safety margins. This is a great advantage and ensures that a process will be under control if it follows the Six Sigma principle.

3.3.4   Multivariate Statistical Process Control

The methods for SPC discussed so far are based on the analysis of one outcome variable at a time (i.e., univariate statistics). However, the quality of food products depends on a whole set of various characteristics. Food quality is, as discussed at the beginning of this chapter, a multivariate property. However, for multivariate systems

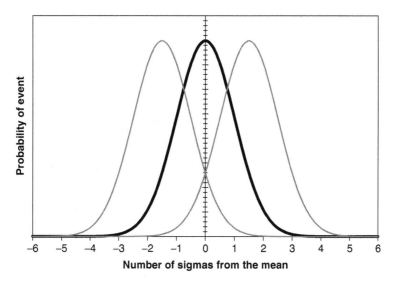

Fig. 3.2 The term "Six Sigma process" is based on statistical theory about the normal distribution. If the lower and upper specification limits are six σ (sigma is the standard deviation of the statistical population), the probability of items failing to meet specifications are extremely low, even if the expected mean of the process shifts (as illustrated by *gray curves*)

there is the obvious constraint of only having two or three dimensions in which to depict patterns graphically. The multivariate statistical method called principal component analysis (PCA) is therefore frequently used in the development of multivariate SPC (Martin et al. 1999). In short, it is a mathematical procedure that uses an orthogonal (i.e., no correlation) transformation to convert a set of observations of possibly correlated variables into a set of values of linearly uncorrelated variables called principal components. The number of principal components is less than or equal to the number of original variables. This transformation is defined in such a way that the first principal component has the largest possible variance (that is, accounts for as much of the variability in the data as possible), and each succeeding component in turn has the highest variance possible under the constraint that it must be orthogonal to (i.e., uncorrelated with) the preceding components. PCA is sensitive to the relative scaling of the original variables. It is therefore common in many applications where it is necessary to do some sort of standardization of the original variables to be on the same scale and at equal variance (e.g., Johnson and Wichern 2007). The statistical properties of PCA will be further discussed in Chap. 5.

In a score plot from PCA the values obtained from the principal component to each sample is plotted as a scatterplot. A schematic score plot to be used in multivariate statistical process control is illustrated in Fig. 3.3 with indicated warning limits. Each axis represents a principal component. It is most common to plot the first two components. Provided the operating conditions remain relatively constant, the scores should continue to lie within the same region of the plot. If some deterioration

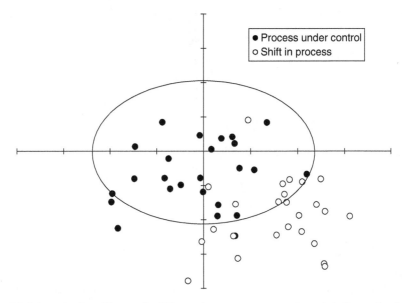

Fig. 3.3 Schematic plot to illustrate the difference between a process under statistical control and after a shift in the process as seen in a score plot from PCA. The *circle* is the estimated warning limits

of performance occurs, then the variability of the process data will change and the scores will start to drift and begin to appear elsewhere. Control limits may be applied in multivariate analysis just as in univariate analysis. These control limits are generally elliptical if used on score plots derived from PCA.

The control limits in multivariate SPC must be based upon a reference data set. The radius of the control limits is typically based on the method of the Mahalanobis or Hotelling T^2 distance. Even though the interpretation of score plots follows many of the same principles as for univariate control charts (Love 2007), it is often more difficult to relate to specific characteristics of a process. Both the statistical method of PCA and estimation limits in score plots are more complex than for univariate analysis. The relationship between the original measurements and the results from PCA may not always be straightforward. Crucial quality characteristics may therefore be preferably assessed using univariate approaches.

3.4 Statistical Assessment of Sensory Data

3.4.1 Methods in Sensory Evaluation

There are three main methods used in sensory evaluation: discrimination tests, descriptive analysis, and hedonic testing (Lawless and Heymann 2010). Sensory science differentiates also between analytical and consumer testing. Statistically,

Table 3.1 Main methods used in sensory evaluation (Partly adopted from Lawless and Heymann 2010)

Main method	Question of interest and purpose
Discrimination testing	Are products perceptibly different in any way? Determine whether there is a detectable difference between products
Descriptive analysis	How do products differ in specific sensory characteristics? Such analysis is widely used in the assessment of different sensory characteristics
Hedonic testing	How well are products liked or which products are preferred? Often connected to consumer testing to evaluate products

the same principles hold for both analytical and consumer testing, but consumer testing may induce biases that are more difficult to control and detect. A representation of the different classes of test methods in sensory evaluation is given in Table 3.1.

The simplest sensory test from a statistical point of view is to detect if there exist any differences between products. One can apply the basis principles of statistical tests presented in Chap. 2 based on the statistical property of the variable describing the sensory outcome data (e.g., numerical or categorical) and whether there exist any dependencies between data (e.g., clustered observation within the same sensory panelist). Discrimination testing is usually based on counting right or wrong answers according to a test setup. From this it follows that statistical analyses are often based on frequencies and proportions. Common methods for discrimination testing include the triangle, duo-trio, and paired comparison procedures. In Box 3.1 the methodological setup of these tests with examples of statistical analyses are given.

Descriptive analyses are methods that quantify intensities in different sensory characteristics of a product. These methods are also sometimes referred to as product flavor or taste profiles. A multivariate statistical approach is very often used in the assessment of descriptive sensory analysis.

Hedonic sensory tests attempt to quantify the degree of liking or disliking of a product. Table 3.2 presents an example of a nine-point hedonic test scale.

3.4.2   Statistical Assessment of Differences Between Foods

The basis of statistical tests is whether to reject the null hypothesis of no difference or effect or accept the null hypothesis. The significance level is then set to avoid the so-called Type I error as discussed previously. In sensory assessment as in all other types of measurements, the type of statistical analysis or test must be chosen based on the nature of the data. If discrimination tests involve choices and counting the number of correct responses as in the triangle test, the statistics are usually derived from a binominal distribution or those designed for proportions. Conversely, for most scaled data, parametric statistics appropriate to normally distributed and

Box 3.1 Common methods for discrimination testing are paired comparison, duo-trio test, and the triangle test. Since the outcome is whether samples are selected, binomial (or chi-squared) tests are applicable as shown in the examples

Type of discrimination test in sensory analysis	Example of experimental study set-up	Example of statistical analysis of data
Paired comparison	Task: Select the sweetest sample (735) (511)	Total number of participants = 50 Participants that selected sample 735 = 30 Participants that selected sample 511 = 20 Binomial test if probability of sample 735 = 0.5 give P-value = 0.203. Common conclusion: No statistical significant difference in sweetness
Duo-trio Test	Task: Select which sample that matches the reference sample (Ref) (Ref) (275) (317)	Total number of participants = 150 Participants that selected sample 735 = 90 Participants that selected sample 511 = 60 Binomial test if probability of sample 275 = 0.5 give P-value = 0.018. Common conclusion: Statistical significant difference between samples 275 and 317 on their matching with reference sample.
Triangle Test	Task: Select the sample that is most different (587)(497)(297) Investigator knows that e.g. sample 497 is the different one and samples 578 and 297 are equal.	Total number of participants = 100 Participants that selected sample 587 = 29 Participants that selected sample 497 = 43 Participants that selected sample 297 = 28 Binomial test if probability of sample 497 = 0.33 give P-value = 0.027. Common conclusion: Statistical significant difference for sample 497 compared with the two similar samples

Table 3.2 The nine-point hedonic scale developed by Peryam and Pilgrim (1957) that is used extensively for acceptance testing. Scale points were chosen to represent equal psychological intervals

Nine-point hedonic scale
Like extremely
Like very much
Like moderately
Like slightly
Neither like nor dislike
Dislike slightly
Dislike moderately
Dislike very much
Dislike extremely

continuous data, such as means, standard deviations, t-tests, or analysis of variance, are appropriate. If the assumption of normal distribution is not valid, then nonparametric tests such as Mann–Whitney or Kruskal–Wallis to compare, respectively, two or more independent groups may be more appropriate. For paired comparisons the Wilcoxon signed-rank test may be used; if there are several sets of grouped data, such as for ranking within a judge, the Friedman test is commonly applied (e.g., Gacula et al. 2009).

3.4.3   *Statistical Assessment of Similarities Between Foods*

The classic goal with statistical analyses and tests is to assess differences by rejecting the null hypothesis of no difference. This is based on statistical-mathematical theory about probabilities on whether observed differences are due to coincidence or representative of an underlying real difference. However, food scientists do not always perform sensory analysis to detect a difference. Often, change in a manufacturing process or the use of ingredients is done to reduce cost, but on the assumption that no difference will occur in the perceived sensory quality of the food product. This is a somewhat unclear situation compared to testing differences. It is impossible to prove that two different samples are exactly equal, i.e., statistically proving the null hypothesis of no difference is not possible. One can only accept or reject the null hypothesis of no difference – not prove that it is true according to statistical theory. Finding no significant difference from a simple discrimination test is not a proof of similarity, noninferiority, or equivalence.

Food scientists may, while statistically assessing that products are similar, draw knowledge from comparable work in medical statistics (Cleophas and Zwinderman 2012; D'Agostino et al. 2003; Snapinn 2000). Noninferiority and equivalence constitute an area of medicine that is attracting increasing interest. It may be difficult to develop pharmaceuticals or treatments that are "better" with respect to the main outcome variables such as life expectancy or key metabolic markers. However, the goal must rather be to develop treatments with an equivalent or at least a noninferior effect on the main outcome but be beneficial in terms of cost or unwanted side effects.

The statistical methods of noninferiority or equivalence testing are in their technicalities not essentially different from discrimination testing. The "difficult" part is determining how much difference or inferiority is acceptable to still regard the samples as equivalent or noninferior. It is tempting and intuitive to want no difference at all, but this is not very realistic and, more crucially, not possible within the framework of statistical theory. Some degree of difference must be accepted to still be able to draw the conclusion that samples are equal. The narrower this acceptable difference, the more samples are needed! Figure 3.4 outlines the principle of statistical inference (reject null hypothesis at significant p-value), noninferiority, and similarity testing. Again, the "difficult" part is to specify in advance the limits of no sensorily relevant difference, i.e., the δ in Fig. 3.4.

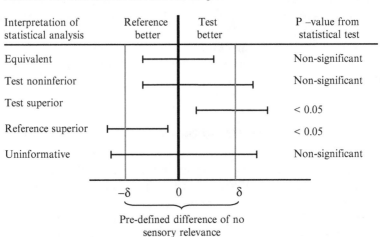

This line ├──────┤ is the width of a 95% confidence interval from a statistical test between reference and test samples

Fig. 3.4 An illustration of the principle behind statistical test of difference, noninferiority, and equivalence

3.5 Statistical Assessment of Shelf Life

3.5.1 Shelf Life and Product Quality

Microbiological, (bio)chemical, physical, and sensory characteristics are all important in the definition of food quality. However, these characteristics change and are strongly affected by storage. Extensive storage time or suboptimal storage conditions reduce food quality and consumer acceptance. Shelf life is therefore an important part of food quality and relevant for statistical analysis. It is the length of time that foods, beverages, pharmaceutical drugs, chemicals, and many other perishable items are given before they are considered unsuitable for sale, use, or consumption. In some regions, a "best before," "use by," or freshness date is required on packaged perishable foods. Shelf life is the recommended amount of time to store products, during which the defined quality of a specified proportion of the goods remains acceptable under expected (or specified) conditions of distribution, storage, and display (e.g., Steele 2004).

Shelf life and stability during storage are important quality characteristics for many foods. Food packaging, distribution, and retail should be optimized to preserve the integrity of a food with its structural, chemical, microbiological, and sensory characteristics in mind. For many foods, their microbiological aspects will determine their shelf life. Sensory tests may also be applicable for many foodstuffs and be closely linked to microbiological or (bio)chemical changes taking place during storage. Sensory shelf-life testing may employ discriminatory, descriptive, or affective testing.

It is common to differentiate between shelf life and expiration date. The former relates to food quality, the latter to food safety. A product that has passed its shelf life might still be safe, but its quality is no longer guaranteed. In most food stores, shelf life is maximized by using stock rotation, which involves moving products with the earliest sell-by date to the front of the shelf, meaning that most shoppers will pick them up first and, thus, get them out of the store. This is important because some stores can be fined for selling out-of-date products, and most if not all will have to mark such products down as wasted, leading to a loss of profit. Exposure to light and heat, transmission of gases (including humidity), mechanical stresses, and contamination by microorganisms may all influence shelf life.

3.5.2   Detection of Shelf Life

Depending on how samples are stored and depending on test times, several options exist for shelf-life tests (e.g., Robertson 2006). The simplest approach is to take batches of the product, store them under normal conditions, and test them at various intervals. For products with a long shelf life, this is not a very efficient approach and may be biased by panels drifting in their criteria over time. A more appropriate design could be to store products at different production times and subsequently test the various samples of different ages at the same time. This could minimize drift in sensory criteria, but it is still very time consuming for products with long shelf lives. A variation on this is to store the product under conditions that essentially stop all aging processes, for example, at very low temperatures. Then products are pulled from the optimal storage conditions at different times and allowed to age at normal temperatures. Another variation of this procedure is to allow products to age for different times and then place them in the optimal storage conditions, pulling everything out of storage at the test date. This is only possible where such storage conditions, e.g., freezing, do not substantially alter product characteristics.

3.5.3   Statistical Assessment of Shelf Life: Food Survival Analysis

When does a product fail as a result of going beyond its shelf life? There are two main criteria for food product failure: (1) a cutoff point on a critical descriptive attribute (e.g., microbial growth) or (2) consumer data/sensory analysis when the product is rejected as unacceptable. Product failure is in statistical terms often a binary property (an all-or-none phenomenon), and decreased sensory attributes such as falling acceptability of increasing proportions of consumer are in statistical terms more continuous. Since product failure is binary, statistical models as logistic regression may be used. The time aspect is a crucial part of shelf life in product failure. Statistical analysis of time to an event (i.e., shelf life until product failure) is statistically usually performed by survival analysis (Kleinbaum and Klein 2005;

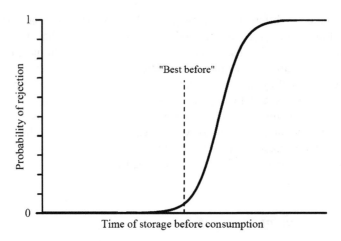

Fig. 3.5 A survival function to be used in the assessment of shelf life based on the probability of consumers' accepting a product beyond a certain storage time. The function is based on the mathematical properties of logistic regression

Aalen et al. 2008), which is a branch of statistics used extensively in clinical studies, epidemiology, biology, and sociology, among others.

Hough et al. (2003) reviewed the use of survival analysis in sensory shelf-life studies. It was pointed out that common sensory experiments produce censored data. That is, for any batch that has failed, we only know that the time of failure was in some interval between the last test and the current test. Similarly, for a batch that has not failed at the final interval, we only know that its failure time is sometime after that final test. So the data are censored and the survival function can be estimated using maximum-likelihood techniques. The survival function was defined as the probability of consumers accepting a product beyond a certain storage time. A schematic survival function based on a logistic regression model is shown in Fig. 3.5.

References

Aalen O, Borgan Ø, Gjessing H (2008) Survival and event history analysis: a process point of view. Springer, New York

Bergman B, Klefsjö B (1994) Quality from consumer needs to customer satisfaction. Studentlitteratur AB, Lund

Cleophas TJ, Zwinderman AH (2012) Equivalence testing, 5th edn, Statistics applied to clinical studies. Springer, Dordrecht

D'Agostino RB Sr, Massaro JM, Sullivan LM (2003) Non-inferiority trials: design concepts and issues – the encounters of academic consultants in statistics. Stat Med 22:169–186. doi:10.1002/sim.1425

Deming WE (1982) Out of the crisis. MIT Press, Cambridge

Gacula MC Jr, Singh J, Bi J, Altan S (2009) Statistical methods in food and consumer research, 2nd edn. Academic, Burlington

Hough G, Langohr K, Gómez G, Curia A (2003) Survival analysis applied to sensory shelf life of foods. J Food Sci 68:359–362. doi:10.1111/j.1365-2621.2003.tb14165.x

Johnson RA, Wichern DW (2007) Applied multivariate statistical analysis, 6th edn. Pearson Prentice Hall, Upper Saddle River

Kleinbaum DG, Klein M (2005) Survival analysis: a self-learning text, 2nd edn. Springer, New York

Lawless HT (1995) Dimensions of quality: a critique. Food Qual Prefer 6:191–196

Lawless HT, Heymann H (2010) Sensory evaluation of food: principles and practices, 2nd edn. Springer, New York

Love J (2007) Statistical process control. In: Process automation handbook. A guide to theory and practice. Springer, New York

Martin EB, Morris AJ, Kiparissides C (1999) Manufacturing performance enhancement through multivariate statistical process control. Annu Rev Control 23:35–44. doi:10.1016/S1367-5788(99)90055-X

McDowell I (2006) Measuring health: a guide to rating scales and questionnaires, 3rd edn. Oxford University Press, Oxford

Naikan VNA (2008) Statistical process control. In: Handbook of performability engineering. Springer, New York

Oakland JS (2007) Statistical process control, 6th edn. Butterworth-Heinemann, Oxford

Peryam DR, Pilgrim FJ (1957) Hedonic scale method of measuring food preference. Food Technol 11:9–14

Robertson GL (2006) Food packaging, principles and practice, 2nd edn. CRC/Taylor and Francis, Boca Raton

Snapinn SM (2000) Noninferiority trials. Curr Control Trials Cardiovasc Med 1:19–21. doi:10.1186/cvm-1-1-019

Steele R (ed) (2004) Understanding and measuring the shelf-life of food. Woodhead, Cambridge

Tennant G (2001) Six Sigma: SPC and TQM in manufacturing and services. Gower, Aldershot

The American Society for Quality (2012) Quality glossary – Q. http://asq.org/glossary/q.html. Accessed 1 May 2012

Wikipedia (2012) Food quality. http://en.wikipedia.org/wiki/Food_quality. Accessed 1 May 2012

Chapter 4
Nutritional Epidemiology and Health Effects of Foods

Abstract The health effects of foods are causing ongoing debates and sometimes controversies. However, results should always be based on the principles underlying clinical and epidemiological research. Important study designs are outlined with special emphasis on case-control, cohort, and intervention studies. Multiple regression models are important in epidemiological studies. However, interpretation depends on a fundamental knowledge of exposure, confounders, and intermediate effects, as will be schematically shown.

Keywords Epidemiology • Case control • Cohort • Confounder

4.1 Food: The Source of Health and Disease

Few areas within food science and nutrition cause such controversies and debates as how foods influence our health and risk of disease. The controversies may sometimes – from a scientific point of view – be somewhat tabloid in their format and message. Claims about specific food products or nutritional components on the risk of cancer, heart disease, and even psychological factors make the headlines. However, it should be beyond doubt that what we eat and drink plays a fundamental role in our health and well-being. While lack of energy and poor nutrition were once a major challenge – and unfortunately still are in many parts of the world – the present focus in developed countries is now more on excess energy, obesity, and how foods contribute to chronic lifestyle diseases like, for example, cardiovascular disease and diabetes. Nutrition, food consumption, and a healthy body mass index (BMI) are closely related to lifestyle as well as socioeconomic factors (e.g., reviews by Darmon and Drewnowski 2008; McAllister et al. 2009; Wang and Beydoun 2007). The close connection between nutrition and food consumption on the one hand and lifestyle and other health issues on the other, one's lifelong "exposure" to food, and the complexity associated with assessing both food intake and its health

A.H. Pripp, *Statistics in Food Science and Nutrition*, SpringerBriefs in Food, Health, and Nutrition, DOI 10.1007/978-1-4614-5010-8_4,
© Springer Science+Business Media New York 2013

effects make nutritional epidemiology a challenging field of research (Michels 2003). To draw sound scientific results for public recommendation, a solid understanding of epidemiological principles and statistical method is paramount.

It is both difficult, and often unethical, to randomly allocate individuals on particular diets for a long time. Therefore, our present knowledge of nutrition is often based on observational studies. Many studies have shown a preventive effect against coronary heart disease of a diet high in polyunsaturated fats and an increased risk related to the intake of trans fats and saturated fats (Stampfer et al. 2000). The risk of type 2 diabetes has also been linked to type of diet and BMI (Hu et al. 2001). Much remains unknown and controversies continue unabated regarding the effects of diet on cancer (Ferguson 2010a) with claimed preventive effects of certain fibers (Roberton et al. 1990, 1991) and probiotic bacteria (Orrhage et al. 1994), and investigators continue to examine the role of mutagens from meat (Ferguson 2010b; Zheng and Lee 2009). With the application of more advanced biostatistical methods such as factor analysis, principal component analysis, cluster analysis, and, not least, structural equation modeling, patterns of diet and lifestyle choices may be better explored in aggregate. Nutrition, food choices, and diet are seldom factors that are isolated from other health and lifestyle considerations.

4.2   Epidemiological Principles and Designs

4.2.1   Clinical and Epidemiological Research Strategies

Clinical and epidemiological research that involves human participants and may result in public health recommendations should be based on clear strategies and objectives. Schematically, clinical and epidemiological research can be divided into four strategies: diagnostic, prognostic, therapeutic, and etiological (Fig. 4.1).

Such a division in research strategy is very useful both for assessing study design and for appropriate statistical analysis. Diagnostic research involves studies that analyze how well methods – both clinical and laboratory – identify a correct diagnosis. This strategy is not very common in nutritional and diet research, even though a correct diagnosis is important for the identification of outcomes. Prognostic research aims to predict future outcomes for patients. Risk scores developed from the Framingham heart study include nutritional aspects such as BMI. Therapeutic research assesses how different treatments affect outcomes. It is very common to base such research on results from randomized clinical trials. The longtime "exposure" of diet, difficulty in sticking to a specified diet, and ethical considerations may limit this strategy in nutritional research. However, for specific nutritional compounds and supplements, the therapeutic research strategy is very important. Examples of randomized diet studies are those with probiotic lactic acid bacteria to prevent or treat diarrheatic diseases (e.g., Parvez et al. 2006) and the therapeutic effects of bioactive compounds in foods to lower blood pressure (e.g., Pripp 2008).

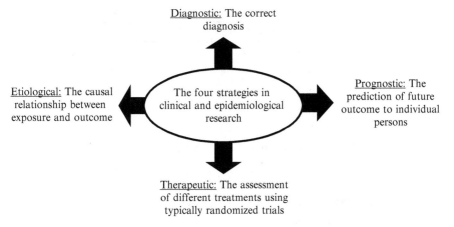

Fig. 4.1 Diagnostic, prognostic, therapeutic, or etiological: the four strategies in clinical and epidemiological research

All of these have a therapeutic research strategy and are based on results from randomized clinical trials. Last but not least – and perhaps most important in diet and nutritional research – is the etiological strategy. This includes studies that claim to assess (causal) relationships between exposure and outcome. Many observational studies in food and nutrition have an etiological objective. They assess how diets affect health issues and claim, to a different degree, that such relationships are causal and not only observed associations.

4.2.2 Clinical and Epidemiological Study Designs

Having an excellent research objective and idea is only half the battle. The actual study must also be conducted! It is then important to use the most appropriate study design. The main categories of clinical and epidemiological study designs are summarized in Table 4.1.

A correlation or ecological study uses data from entire populations to compare disease frequency among different groups during the same period of time or among the same population at different times. Thus, results are based on summarized data (e.g., averages, proportions) from entire populations and do not contain individual subject data. An example of an ecological study in food science and nutrition is the consumption of different dietary fats and health status in regions that are based on region-specific data and not individuals (Moussavi et al. 2008).

Case reports or case series are based on data from a few individual patients. They are of limited interest from a statistical point of view since they are based on results from a small number of selected subjects, but they can provide information about unknown effects of exposure and diseases. Typically, this might include reports of toxicity or the clinical effects of nutritional compounds or diets for certain patients.

Table 4.1 The main clinical and epidemiological study designs

Main clinical and epidemiological study designs	
Randomized clinical trials	
Cohort studies (with longitudinal data)	
Case-control studies	Increased degree of causal interpretation
Cross-sectional studies and surveys	
Case reports and case series	
Ecological studies (no subject specific data)	

Case-control study: Selection into study on basis of disease status

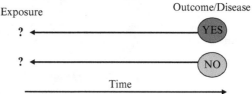

Cohort study: Selection into study on basis of exposure status

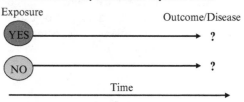

Intervention study: Prospective study in which exposure is (randomly) allocated by investigator

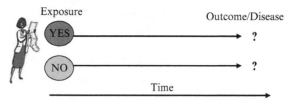

Fig. 4.2 Illustration of study designs of case-control, cohort, and intervention studies. These are all analytical designs frequently used in clinical and epidemiological research

Cross-sectional studies are "snapshots" in time. They provide information on the exposure and outcome of individuals assessed simultaneously and are frequently used to assess the prevalence of diseases. Since they do not contain longitudinal or follow-up data on the individual level, it is from a logical point of view only possible to assess association and not causal relationships. For example, it is – strictly methodologically speaking – not possible, without longitudinal data, to say whether eating chocolate increases a person's BMI or whether an increased BMI causes higher consumption of chocolate.

Case-control, cohort, and intervention studies are often referred to as analytical study designs in clinical and epidemiological research (Fig. 4.2). In a case-control study subjects are selected and included in the study on the basis of disease status. Logistic regression is frequently used to statistically analyze case-control studies. In a (longitudinal) cohort study, subjects are selected and included in the study based on exposure status. If a cohort is studied retrospectively, it can be referred to as a historic cohort study. The study design differs from a cross-sectional study by the fact that data are recorded over time for the subjects (e.g., Rothman 2002). In an intervention study, the exposure is allocated (often randomly) to participants by an investigator. Randomized clinical trials are types of intervention studies used extensively in clinical research and especially in the assessment of new pharmaceuticals.

4.3 Methods to Assess Food Intake

A fundamental challenge in nutritional epidemiology is to obtain valid and reliable data on both exposure and outcome in relation to diet. Various methods exist to obtain diet-related data. Food consumption can be assessed on an overall level based on statistics on food production, import, and export. This produces data on group or regional levels but does not provide information on individual subjects.

To obtain data on the individual level, food-frequency questionnaires have been extensively used to gather subject-specific data on diet. Participants are asked to answer questions on how often within a given time frame they have eaten certain food items. A typical example is the question, used in the Oslo Health Study, of how often a person drinks semi-skimmed milk? Answers included Seldom/never, 1–6 glasses per week, 1 glass per day, 2–3 glasses per day, or 4 glasses or more per day.

Another related method is a 24-h diet interview. The objective is not to obtain an average expression of diet but rather specific consumption information over the last 24 h. It usually takes considerable effort to transform the information obtained from the interview into variables and data to be used in statistical analysis. A diet historical interview is another approach that asks participants what they usually consume. This interview can be regarded as a more open approach than the food-frequency questionnaire. It is also a challenge to transform observations from the interview into usable variables and data for statistical analysis. Diet registration is a method whereby each participant registers what is consumed. The registration can be rather open where subjects make notes about their diet (Hjartåker and Veierød 2007).

All methods based on interviews or questionnaires are prone to errors and recall biases. Therefore, biological markers are often used in medical and clinical studies and play a role in nutritional research. Such markers can provide objective data and are not prone to subjective errors and biases. However, biological and metabolic markers may be influenced by subject characteristics such as age, gender, and other diseases. Patterns of fatty acids or karotenoids in the blood have been used to assess intake of fats or vegetables, respectively. Ideally, biological markers should be validated and compared with data from interviews or food-frequency questionnaires (Baylin et al. 2002).

4.4   Epidemiological Use of Multiple Regression Models

Confounding, effect modification (interaction), and intermediate effects in causal pathways are important concepts in epidemiology. The statistical method of choice is often a multiple regression model. Depending on the outcome (dependent variable), linear, logistic, Poisson, Cox, or other main types of generalized linear models may be applied. Multiple regression models are used extensively in epidemiological research. It is often the statistical method of choice for assessing confounder effects, effect modification (interaction), or intermediate effects in many observational studies. The use and interpretation of such models should be viewed in relation to the study design and epidemiological principles.

To illustrate these concepts, let us assume that we have a longitudinal study with two indentified cohorts. One cohort follows a diet low in carbohydrates and the other follows a so-called regular diet. Since this is not a randomized trial, there might be other differences between the two groups in addition to type of diet. Low-carbohydrate diets are from time to time popularized as a healthy, more biologically natural and efficient method for weight control, but the scientific evidence of such claims has been disputed by other nutritional experts (Bravata et al. 2003). Let us further assume that the outcome after a given follow–up time is BMI. Other observed variables, in addition to diet and BMI, that may be of importance are assumed to be the degree of physical activity (ACTIVITY), average calorie intake (INTAKE), age of participant (AGE), and the gender of the participants (GENDER) (Table 4.2).

4.4.1   Adjusting for Confounders

Confounding is a rather common term, even frequently used in everyday language, and often without a strict understanding of its statistical and epidemiological meaning. A confounding variable is sometimes referred to as a hidden or lurking variable. It is defined as a variable that correlates with both the exposure (CARBODIET in our example) and outcome (BMI in our example) variable. The causal pathway should only be in one direction for a confounder – it is from the confounder to the exposure and outcome variable (Box 4.1). This means that changes in the confounder affect the exposure and outcome variable, but not the other way around. For example, age may affect the probability of choosing a low-carb diet (exposure) and the BMI (outcome) of an individual. However, changes in the BMI or choosing a low-carb diet does not affect age (even though some people tend to behave as if it did!).

Table 4.2 Description of variables to illustrate interpretation of multiple regression models in an assumed epidemiological cohort study

Variable	Description of variable
CARBODIET	If the subject is on a low-carbohydrate diet or on a regular diet, i.e., the exposure of interest
GENDER	Participant's gender
AGE	Participant's age in years
INTAKE	Participant's daily calorie intake
ACTIVITY	Degree of participant's physical activity
BMI	Participant's body mass index after following the (self)-chosen diet for a given time, i.e., outcome of interest

Box 4.1 Causal relationship between exposure, confounders, and outcome and the interpretation of relevant regression models

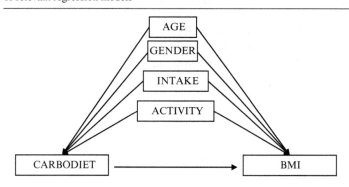

Selected regression models

Interpretation of the regression coefficient to the exposure variable CARBODIET

$BMI_i = \beta_0 + \beta_1 \cdot CARBODIET + \varepsilon_i$

Model 1: The coefficient β_1 is called the unadjusted or crude estimate, i.e. the observed difference between the two diets on BMI

$BMI_i = \beta_0 + \beta_1 \cdot CARBODIET$
$+ \beta_2 \cdot AGE + \beta_3 \cdot GENDER$
$+ \beta_4 \cdot INTAKE + \beta_4 \cdot ACTIVITY + \varepsilon_i$

Model 2: The coefficient β_1 is called the adjusted estimate, i.e. the estimated difference between chosen type of diet on BMI given that ACTIVITY, INTAKE, AGE, and GENDER were equal in the two diet groups and these confounders would then not influence the exposure effect.

There are two methodological strategies to account for confounders. One strategy is to account for them in the design phase of a study, as with randomized trials, whereas the other is to account for them in the statistical analysis using, for example, multiple regression models. Matching participants (or groups of participants) on possible confounders such as age and gender is another strategy, but that involves taking into account confounders both in the design and analysis phases of a study. A matched design should be analyzed using statistical methods for matched data as, for example, a paired *t*-test. Generally speaking, matching on variables that may be measured easily like AGE and GENDER complicates both the design and statistical analysis of a study. Therefore, the author does not recommend matching on variables that can be measured. It is more efficient to control these by using multiple regression models.

If ACTIVITY, INTAKE, AGE, and GENDER are confounders in relation to the effect of CARBODIET on BMI, then the statistical approach to adjusting for their confounding effect is to include them as independent variables in a multiple regression model. Thus, the coefficient β_1 from the simple regression model with only CARBODIET in relation to BMI (model 1 in Box 4.1) is the actual observed difference between the cohorts on a low-carb versus a regular diet. The coefficient of CARBODIET (also denoted β_1) in relation to BMI from the multiple regression model (model 2 in Box 4.1) is the so-called confounder-adjusted estimate between low-carb versus regular diet in relation to BMI. This estimate is the statistically adjusted estimated difference in BMI between the diet groups given that the distribution of ACTIVITY, INTAKE, AGE, and GENDER was equal between the two cohorts. If the distribution of confounders was equal between the exposure groups, then they would not influence the estimated effect of CARBODIET on BMI. Thus, the name *adjusted estimate*.

4.4.2 Assessment of Effect Modification (Interaction)

While confounding variables are a source of problems we would like to eliminate in the design or analysis phase of a study, effect modification or interaction is an interesting effect that should be carefully studied and reported. It is present if the magnitude of the relationship between the exposure (CARBODIET in our example) and outcome (BMI in our example) differs in size (is modified) from the level of a third variable called the effect modifier. Effect modification is not the most obvious effect in our example with low-carb or regular diet. For the sake of illustration, one could imagine that a low-carb diet had an effect on BMI for females but not for males. Thus the effect of CARBODIET would be different for males and females. Note: this is different from the independent effect of GENDER. It would be statistically assessed with an interaction term between CARBODIET and GENDER in the multiple regression model. If this term was significant, results could be reported separately for males and females since they would experience different effects of the exposure variable CARBODIET.

From a scientific point of view, effect modification – which we statistically assess with an interaction term in multiple regression models – is exciting. However, both the explanation of effects and their presentation become more complicated. One should therefore be somewhat careful about including interaction terms if one does not "believe" in them. Statistically, there may be several significant interaction terms in a multiple regression model, especially if the number of observations is large. However, the scientific basis of a true and important effect modification may not always be present. One piece of advice is to test for effect modification only on the basis of a sound scientific theory.

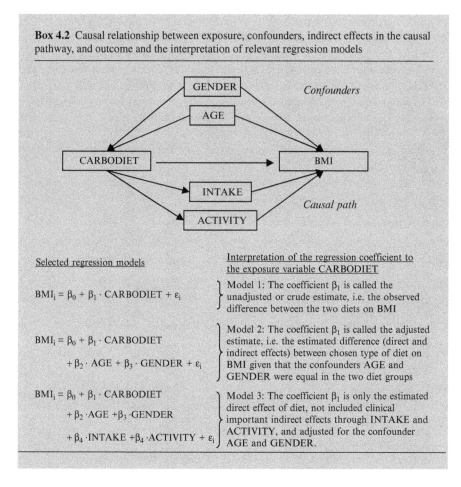

Box 4.2 Causal relationship between exposure, confounders, indirect effects in the causal pathway, and outcome and the interpretation of relevant regression models

Selected regression models	Interpretation of the regression coefficient to the exposure variable CARBODIET
$BMI_i = \beta_0 + \beta_1 \cdot CARBODIET + \varepsilon_i$	Model 1: The coefficient β_1 is called the unadjusted or crude estimate, i.e. the observed difference between the two diets on BMI
$BMI_i = \beta_0 + \beta_1 \cdot CARBODIET$ $+ \beta_2 \cdot AGE + \beta_3 \cdot GENDER + \varepsilon_i$	Model 2: The coefficient β_1 is called the adjusted estimate, i.e. the estimated difference (direct and indirect effects) between chosen type of diet on BMI given that the confounders AGE and GENDER were equal in the two diet groups
$BMI_i = \beta_0 + \beta_1 \cdot CARBODIET$ $+ \beta_2 \cdot AGE + \beta_3 \cdot GENDER$ $+ \beta_4 \cdot INTAKE + \beta_4 \cdot ACTIVITY + \varepsilon_i$	Model 3: The coefficient β_1 is only the estimated direct effect of diet, not included clinical important indirect effects through INTAKE and ACTIVITY, and adjusted for the confounder AGE and GENDER.

4.4.3 Intermediate Variables in the Causal Pathway

There is a large difference in the analysis and interpretation of a variable depending on whether it is a confounder or an intermediate in the causal pathway. It is therefore very important to assess, on the basis of scientific knowledge, whether variables are confounders or intermediates. They might be both, but this, of course, would complicate further analysis and would often require the use of more advanced statistical methods such as structural equation modeling.

Let us assume that ACTIVITY and INTAKE are not confounders, but instead intermediate variables in the causal pathway. Thus, they do not "disturb" the effect of CARBODIET on BMI but, on the contrary, indirectly cause an effect by CARBODIET on BMI. Our causal model is now that CARBODIET cause changes in both ACTIVITY and INTAKE, which then indirectly cause an effect on BMI in addition to the direct effect of CARBODIET (see Box 4.2 for an illustration of causal pathways).

The simple linear regression model with only CARBODIET (model 1 in Box 4.2) is still the observed mean difference in BMI between diet cohorts. However, in the multiple linear regression model with CARBODIET, ACTIVITY, INTAKE, AGE, and GENDER, the CARBODIET coefficient is now the estimated direct effect of type of diet on BMI (model 3 in Box 4.2). This does not take into account the clinically important indirect effects of ACTIVITY and INTAKE. If we assume that these indirect effects are important, but the direct effect is negligible, then CARBODIET will be insignificant in this model. However, in a simplified model with CARBODIET, AGE, and GENDER (model 2 in Box 4.2), the coefficient will be significant and serve as an estimate of the true causal effect of CARBODIET including both the (assumed negligible) direct and highly relevant indirect effect through change in ACTIVITY and INTAKE.

References

Baylin A, Kabagambe EK, Siles X, Campos H (2002) Adipose tissue biomarkers of fatty acid intake. Am J Clin Nutr 76:750–757

Bravata DM, Sanders L, Huang J, Krumholz HM, Olkin I, Gardner CD, Bravata DM (2003) Efficacy and safety of low-carbohydrate diets: a systematic review. JAMA 289:1837–1850. doi:10.1001/jama.289.14.1837

Darmon N, Drewnowski A (2008) Does social class predict diet quality. Am J Clin Nutr 87:1107–1117

Ferguson LR (2010a) Dietary influence on mutagenesis – where is this field going. Environ Mol Mutagen 51:909–918. doi:10.1002/em.20594

Ferguson LR (2010b) Meat and cancer. Meat Sci 84:308–313. doi:10.1016/j.meatsci.2009.06.032

Hjartåker A, Veierød MB (2007) Ernæringsforskning. In: Laake P, Hjartåker A, Thelle DS, Veierød MB (eds) Epidemiologiske og kliniske forskningsmetoder. Gyldendal Norsk Forlag, Oslo

Hu FB, Manson JE, Stampfer MJ, Colditz G, Liu S, Solomon CG, Willett WC (2001) Diet, lifestyle, and the risk of type 2 diabetes mellitus in women. N Engl J Med 345:790–797. doi:10.1056/NEJMoa010492

McAllister EJ, Dhurandhar NV, Keith SW, Aronne LJ, Barger J, Baskin M, Benca RM, Biggio J, Boggiano MM, Eisenmann JC, Elobeid M, Fontaine KR, Gluckman P, Hanlon EC, Katzmarzyk P, Pietrobelli A, Redden DT, Ruden DM, Wang C, Waterland RA, Wright SM, Allison DB (2009) Ten putative contributors to the obesity epidemic. Crit Rev Food Sci Nutr 49:868–913. doi:10.1080/10408390903372599

Michels KB (2003) Nutritional epidemiology – past, present, future. Int J Epidemiol 32:486–488. doi:10.1093/ije/dyg216

Moussavi N, Gavino V, Receveur O (2008) Is obesity related to the type of dietary fatty acids? An ecological study. Public Health Nutr 11:1149–1155. doi:10.1017/S1368980007001541

Orrhage K, Sillerstrom E, Gustafsson JA, Nord CE, Rafter J (1994) Binding of mutagenic heterocyclic amines by intestinal and lactic acid bacteria. Mutat Res 311:239–248. doi:10.1016/0027-5107(94)90182-1

Parvez S, Malik KA, Kang SA, Kim HY (2006) Probiotics and their fermented food products are beneficial for health. J Appl Microbiol 100:1171–1185. doi:10.1111/j.1365-2672.2006.02963.x

Pripp AH (2008) Effect of peptides derived from food proteins on blood pressure: a meta-analysis of randomized controlled trials. Food Nutr Res 58:1–9. doi:10.3402/fnr.v52i0.1641

Roberton AM, Ferguson LR, Hollands HJ, Harris PJ (1990) A model system for studying the adsorption of a hydrophobic mutagen to dietary fibre. Mutat Res 244:173–178. doi:10.1016/0165-7992(90)90068-U

Roberton AM, Ferguson LR, Hollands HJ, Harris PJ (1991) Adsorption of a hydrophobic mutagen to five contrasting dietary preparations. Mutat Res 262:195–202. doi:10.1016/0165-7992(91)90022-V

Rothman KJ (2002) Epidemiology: an introduction. Oxford University Press, New York

Stampfer MJ, Hu FB, Manson JE, Rimm EB, Willett WC (2000) Primary prevention of coronary heart disease in women through diet and lifestyle. N Engl J Med 343:16–22. doi:10.1056/NEJM200007063430103

Wang Y, Beydoun MA (2007) The obesity epidemic in the United States – gender, age, socioeconomic, racial/ethnic, and geographic characteristics: a systematic review and meta-regression analysis. Epidemiol Rev 29:6–28. doi:10.1093/epirev/mxm007

Zheng W, Lee SA (2009) Well-done meat intake, heterocyclic amine exposure, and cancer risk. Nutr Cancer 61:437–446. doi:10.1080/01635580802710741

Chapter 5
Application of Multivariate Analysis: Benefits and Pitfalls

Abstract Multivariate statistical methods involve the simultaneous analysis of more than one outcome variable. In applied use, this definition is sometimes relaxed, but it typically includes methods such as principal component analysis, factor analysis, cluster analysis, and partial least-squares regression. Methods based on principal component analysis are frequently encountered in food science, and it is therefore compared with factor analysis, commonly used in biostatistics. The interpretation of results, especially in relation to the original variables, might be challenging, which could represent these methods' weakest link from an applied point of view.

Keywords Principal component analysis • Factor analysis • Chemometrics

5.1 Introduction of Multivariate Statistics in Food Science

Multivariate statistics – in strict statistical terminology – differs from univariate methods in that it involves the simultaneous analysis of more than one outcome (dependent) variable. It includes methods that are relatively frequently used in food science such as, for example, multivariate analysis of variance (MANOVA), principal component analysis (PCA), factor analysis (FA), cluster analysis (CA), and artificial neural networks (ANN). Methods like principal component regression (PCR) and partial least-squares regression (PLSR) with multiple dependent variables have been developed, but they are often denoted as multivariate statistics even when used with one dependent variable. They are used in food science, technology, and nutrition applications in areas such as chemical analysis of food components, clustering of products, spectroscopic analysis and prediction, quantitative structure activity analysis, and sensory analysis, among others (see e.g. reviews by Karoui and Baerdermaeker 2007; Pripp et al. 2005; Tzouros and Arvanitoyannis 2001). Their contribution to food science and technology is substantial with giving new

A.H. Pripp, *Statistics in Food Science and Nutrition*, SpringerBriefs in Food, Health, and Nutrition, DOI 10.1007/978-1-4614-5010-8_5,
© Springer Science+Business Media New York 2013

scientific insight into the complex relationship between biology, technology and consumer perception.

On a personal level, I have always found great scientific interest in and useful applications of these methods in applied statistical analysis within food science, technology and nutrition. However, as a result of my involvement in medical statistics and clinical epidemiology, I have noticed that such multivariate methods seem to be used less often in medical and health research compared to its somewhat frequent use in food science. One exception might be psychological and psychiatric research, but even here there is a tendency to use methods such as FA or structural equations and not methods like PCA or PLSR (Fabrigar et al. 1999; Kahn 2006; Widaman 1993).

Multivariate methods like PCA are sometimes used in settings where they are statistically less suited. The interpretation of results yielded from using methods like PCA or PLSR and especially in relation to the initial measured variables might be challenging and may be these methods' weakest link from an applied point of view.

5.2 Principal Component Analysis or Factor Analysis: When and Where

PCA and (explorative) FA are both variable reduction techniques and sometimes mistakenly regarded as close variants of the same methods. However, there are distinct differences between PCA and FA, both in statistical theory and in their recommended applied uses (Suhr 2009).

5.2.1 What Is Principal Component Analysis?

Methodologically speaking, PCA is first of all a variable reduction technique, often used where variables are highly correlated, that reduces the number of observed variables to a smaller number of principal components, which accounts for the variance of the observed variables. The principal components are retained to account for a maximal amount of variance of observed variables, and all the retained principal components are uncorrelated with each other. Component scores are linear combinations of observed variables weighted by eigenvectors (loadings). They are concerned with explaining the variance–covariance structure through a few linear combinations of initial variables.

To reproduce the total system variability, one must have as many components as there are initial variables. Often much of this variability can be accounted for by a small number of principal components. If so, there is (almost) as much information about the system variability in the few components as there is in the initial variables.

In statistical language, the k principal components can then replace the initial p variables, and the original data set, consisting of n measurements on p variables, is reduced to one consisting of n measurements on k principal components.

To outline the statistical-mathematical difference between PCA and FA, let us assume we have six measured variables. These six variables are denoted X_1, X_2, X_3, X_4, X_5, and X_6. The principal components are those (uncorrelated) linear combinations of X_1, X_2, X_3, X_4, X_5, and X_6 whose variance is as large as possible. If we call the first principal component PC1 and the sixth and last principal component PC6, it can be expressed as the following linear models:

$$PC_1 = \ell_{11}X_1 + \ell_{21}X_2 + \ell_{31}X_3 + \ell_{41}X_4 + \ell_{51}X_5 + \ell_{61}X_6$$
$$PC_2 = \ell_{12}X_1 + \ell_{22}X_2 + \ell_{32}X_3 + \ell_{42}X_4 + \ell_{52}X_5 + \ell_{62}X_6$$
$$PC_3 = \ell_{13}X_1 + \ell_{23}X_2 + \ell_{33}X_3 + \ell_{43}X_4 + \ell_{53}X_5 + \ell_{63}X_6$$
$$PC_4 = \ell_{14}X_1 + \ell_{24}X_2 + \ell_{34}X_3 + \ell_{44}X_4 + \ell_{54}X_5 + \ell_{64}X_6$$
$$PC_5 = \ell_{15}X_1 + \ell_{25}X_2 + \ell_{35}X_3 + \ell_{45}X_4 + \ell_{55}X_5 + \ell_{65}X_6$$
$$PC_6 = \ell_{16}X_1 + \ell_{26}X_2 + \ell_{36}X_3 + \ell_{46}X_4 + \ell_{56}X_5 + \ell_{66}X_6$$

where ℓ is the coefficient multiplied by the initial measured variables in the linear combinations that compose each principal component. These coefficients are usually called loadings. The initial variables are in many applications standardized to, for example, a mean of zero and a standard deviation of one (Z-standardization) to compare the variables on the same unit scale.

In many applications of PCA, it is common to express the data structure through the first few principal components. Let us assume that the first two principal components express the data structure sufficiently. Thus, in our statistical-mathematical notation this can be expressed as

$$PC_1 = \ell_{11}X_1 + \ell_{21}X_2 + \ell_{31}X_3 + \ell_{41}X_4 + \ell_{51}X_5 + \ell_{61}X_6$$
$$PC_2 = \ell_{12}X_1 + \ell_{22}X_2 + \ell_{32}X_3 + \ell_{42}X_4 + \ell_{52}X_5 + \ell_{62}X_6$$

| The two first important ones |

$$PC_3 = \ell_{13}X_1 + \ell_{23}X_2 + \ell_{33}X_3 + \ell_{43}X_4 + \ell_{53}X_5 + \ell_{63}X_6$$
$$PC_4 = \ell_{14}X_1 + \ell_{24}X_2 + \ell_{34}X_3 + \ell_{44}X_4 + \ell_{54}X_5 + \ell_{64}X_6$$
$$PC_5 = \ell_{15}X_1 + \ell_{25}X_2 + \ell_{35}X_3 + \ell_{45}X_4 + \ell_{55}X_5 + \ell_{65}X_6$$
$$PC_6 = \ell_{16}X_1 + \ell_{26}X_2 + \ell_{36}X_3 + \ell_{46}X_4 + \ell_{56}X_5 + \ell_{66}X_6$$

| The remaining ones that is regarded as noise (interpreted as kind of random error) |

The amount of variance explained by each principal component can be denoted by λ. In our illustration with the initial six measured variables we have that

$$\begin{bmatrix} \text{Proportion of total} \\ \text{population variance due to the} \\ \text{kth principal component} \end{bmatrix} = \frac{\lambda_k}{\lambda_1 + \lambda_2 + \lambda_3 + \lambda_4 + \lambda_5 + \lambda_6}$$

If most (for instance, 80–90 %) of the total population variance in the data set can be attributed to the first few components, then these components can "replace" all the originally measured variables without much "loss of information" (see, e.g., Johnson and Wichern 2007 for a comprehensive description of statistical-mathematical theory on PCA). PCA is, as previously mentioned, commonly used for applied data analysis in fields like chemometrics, spectroscopy, image compression, and sensory analysis.

5.2.2 What Is Factor Analysis?

Exploratory FA, on the other hand, is a variable reduction technique that identifies the number of latent constructs and the underlying factor structure of a set of variables. It is based on a hypothesis of an underlying construct, a variable not measured directly. This allows one to describe and identify a number of latent unique constructs (factors) and errors due to an unreliability in measurements. Factors account for common variance in the data. Observed variables are linear combinations of the underlying and unique factors. The essential purpose of FA is to describe, if possible, the covariance relationships among many variables in terms of a few underlying, but unobservable, quantities called factors. In many aspects, compared with PCA, FA has more in common with such statistical methods as regression analysis where the outcome is explained as a model with parameters and with a random error term to account for deviations between the model and what is observed.

An FA is motivated by the following argument. Suppose variables can be grouped by their correlation. That is, all variables within a particular group are highly correlated by themselves but have relatively small correlation with variables in a different group. It is conceivable that each group of variables represents a single underlying construct, or factor, that is responsible for the observed correlation. The primary question in FA is whether the data are consistent with a prescribed structure.

It is often graphically illustrated using circles for factors and squares for observed variables. A two-factor model based on six assumed variables X_1 to X_6 is given in Fig. 5.1. The arrows indicate the "causal" direction. The argument is that the underlying factor, together with random noise/variation, is what makes the observed variable. It is common to standardize the observed variables to a mean of zero and a standard deviation of one by subtracting the mean and divide by the standard deviation (Z-standardize), as is also the case in PCA. FA postulates then that our six observed variables are linearly dependent upon two unobservable common factors, F1 and F2, and six additional sources of variation (ε) called (random) errors or specific factors. In mathematical notation a two-factor model on six initial variables can be written as

Fig. 5.1 Graphical
representation of an assumed
factor analysis model. Two
underlying constructs or
factors (F$_1$ and F$_2$) influence
the six measured variables X_1
to X_6. The first factor, F$_1$, is
assumed to "express" itself
by the observed variables X_1,
X_2, and X_3, and factor F2 is
assumed to "express" itself
by the observed variables X_4,
X_5, and X_6. In addition, all
the observed variables are
influenced by their respective
random error terms ε_1 to ε_6.

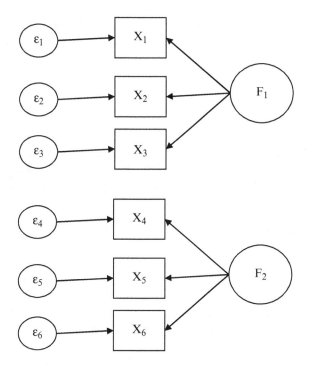

$$X_1 = \mu_1 + \ell_{11}F_1 + \ell_{12}F_2 + \varepsilon_1$$
$$X_2 = \mu_2 + \ell_{21}F_1 + \ell_{22}F_2 + \varepsilon_2$$
$$X_3 = \mu_3 + \ell_{31}F_1 + \ell_{32}F_2 + \varepsilon_3$$
$$X_4 = \mu_4 + \ell_{41}F_1 + \ell_{42}F_2 + \varepsilon_4$$
$$X_5 = \mu_5 + \ell_{51}F_1 + \ell_{52}F_2 + \varepsilon_5$$
$$X_6 = \mu_6 + \ell_{61}F_1 + \ell_{62}F_2 + \varepsilon_6$$

The coefficient ℓ, known as the loadings of the given variable on the specific factor, and the μ and ε are the expected mean and (random) error, respectively, of each variable. In the model in Fig. 5.1, the loadings of factor 2 (F$_2$) are set to zero for the observed variables X_1, X_2, and X_3 and the loadings of factor 1 (F$_1$) are set to zero for the observed variables X_4, X_5, and X_6. If the variables are not standardized, then they can be interpreted as the slope coefficient from the factor on the observed variable. If the variables are standardized to a standard deviation of one and are approximately normally distributed, then the loading may be interpreted as the correlation between the underlying factor and the observed variable. In explorative FA it is very common to use Z-standardized variables to facilitate interpretation across variables. However, each variable is then unit free and *equally important* at the beginning of modeling (see, e.g., the textbook by Johnson and Wichern 2007 for a comprehensive description of statistical-mathematical theory on FA).

5.2.3 Overall Recommendations

PCA has been used extensively in food research in areas like proteomics, sensory science, chromatography, and consumer science, while FA is typically used in medical statistics and especially in psychometrics. Sometimes there is controversy regarding the benefits and disadvantages between the applied uses of these two techniques. An important difference is that FA takes into account the existence of random error for each observed variable, whereas PCA in statistical-mathematical terms does not. In PCA, all the variance in the data, i.e., variance unique to each variable, variance common among variables, and error variance, is treated as one. In contrast, in FA, the goal is to model the shared variance. It has therefore been recommended to use FA when there are theoretical ideas concerning the relationships between variables, whereas PCA should be used if the goal of the research is to explore patterns in the data or merely perform variable reduction to use in prediction models. FA may also be more appropriate where random error might be important for the measured variables. The random error could be substantial for items in questionnaires used in psychometric research, but also scores in sensory panels and from consumers may be influenced by random error. Strictly methodologically speaking, this is an argument for using FA instead of PCA on sensory data.

A personal view: PCA may be the method of choice if the goal is merely data reduction, prediction using PCR (or the related PLSR method), or exploration of the data structure without a view to developing a model based on the relationship between variables. It should, however, be limited to variables where random error might be negligible. (Exploratory) FA might be more suited to exploring underlying patterns between variables for the purpose of developing models, interpreting underlying effects, and combining items into a factor or when the random error of each variable might be substantial.

To illustrate the relationship between the population-based properties of variables given by the expected mean, standard deviation, and correlation structure and how a typical random sample is given these population characteristics as well as the sample's analysis using PCA and FA, a simulated example is given in Box 5.1. It might be difficult to explore the original population characteristics of the six variables given only the estimated loadings from FA or PCA.

Box 5.1   A simulated example to show the relationship between the statistical properties in the population, a random sample from this population, and analysis with PCA or FA of the 20 samples. These data are also used for descriptive plots in Fig. 2.1

The properties of the statistical population, i.e. the statistical truth.

Expected statistical properties of six normal distributed variables

Variable	Expected mean (μ)	Expected st.dev. (σ)
X1	0	1
X2	2	2
X3	4	1
X4	6	2
X5	8	1
X6	10	2

Expected correlation matrix

	X1	X2	X3	X4	X5	X6
X1	1.0	0.8	-0.8	0	0	0
X2	0.8	1.0	-0.8	0	0	0
X3	-0.8	-0.8	1.0	0	0	0
X4	0	0	0	1.0	0.8	-0.8
X5	0	0	0	0.8	1.0	-0.8
X6	0	0	0	-0.8	-0.8	1.0

A typical random sample from the described statistical population

What you typically would observed if measured 20 samples of these variables

sample	x1	x2	x3	x4	x5	x6
1	3.3	7.5	2.2	4.6	7.5	9.8
2	0.4	2.5	3.6	8.1	9.1	6.8
3	-0.3	3.0	4.1	3.6	6.5	11.1
4	0.6	3.7	3.3	8.4	8.3	8.2
5	2.2	2.9	3.1	6.6	9.6	8.8
6	-0.3	1.3	4.3	8.6	9.4	7.8
7	-0.4	1.5	3.9	6.4	7.9	10.8
8	-2.2	-2.1	5.8	4.1	6.6	12.2
9	0.6	2.1	4.0	6.2	7.7	10.4
10	1.1	5.1	2.4	4.7	7.3	11.6
11	1.0	5.0	2.8	5.2	8.2	10.1
12	-0.4	1.8	4.0	4.1	7.2	11.4
13	-0.8	0.9	4.9	6.8	7.3	9.1
14	-0.8	2.4	4.0	6.3	7.9	8.9
15	-0.8	-0.1	4.5	5.8	6.8	11.2
16	0.8	1.4	3.6	8.0	8.8	8.2
17	1.7	6.2	2.3	8.3	9.0	6.7
18	1.3	4.1	2.6	6.0	7.3	9.1
19	-0.9	1.1	4.6	8.2	8.3	9.7
20	-0.8	1.4	4.3	3.0	5.9	13.3

Results from principal component analysis (PCA) and factor analysis (FA) with two extracted components / factors (with percent explained variance) and with varimax rotation (varimax) of the 20 simulated samples above. All initial variables standardized to mean of zero and standard deviation of one. Loadings with low values were set to zero in the confirmatory factor analysis (CFA)

	PCA		PCA (varimax)		FA		FA (varimax)		CFA	
	PC1 (59%)	PC2 (33%)	PC1 (48%)	PC2 (45%)	F1 (65%)	F2 (35%)	F1 (53%)	F2 (49%)	F1	F2
X1	0.44	-0.33	0.55	0.05	0.82	-0.43	0.90	0.21	0.91	-
X2	0.40	-0.43	0.58	-0.05	0.76	-0.58	0.95	0.06	0.94	-
X3	-0.43	0.38	-0.58	0.00	-0.81	0.52	-0.96	-0.14	-0.99	-
X4	0.32	0.53	-0.11	0.61	0.58	0.74	-0.04	0.94	-	0.92
X5	0.41	0.38	0.06	0.56	0.74	0.52	0.23	0.88	-	0.9
X6	-0.43	-0.37	-0.08	-0.56	-0.78	-0.52	-0.26	-0.90	-	-0.94

5.3　Exploratory Data Analysis

The overall goal of multivariate exploratory data is to perform dimensionality reduction to concentrate information and improve graphical representation. This is useful for enhancing understanding, for conceptualization, and for detecting structures in data. In an unsupervised approach, one does not use class information but tries to find natural groupings and detect possible outliers. This is in contrast to a supervised approach, where one uses known class information to maximize separation and detect the underlying structures of the known classes.

Examples of multivariate exploratory data analysis methods used in food science are PCA, FA, and CA. If there is no underlying model, the PCA or CA may be the methods of choice. Both can detect extreme outliers and indicate underlying patterns. They have been applied in an explorative approach in many subfields within food science and nutrition (Kozak and Scaman 2008). However, PCA is statistically first of all a variable reduction technique and not a method for classification or clustering. Therefore, the question may arise as to whether it is methodologically a very efficient approach for unsupervised classification and whether CA should instead be the preferred method.

Is it important to first examine data with basic explorative techniques such as box plots and scatterplots, or is it feasible to use immediately the aforementioned multivariate techniques for explorative data analysis? The author's personal experience in applied statistics suggests several arguments for using basic explorative graphical techniques and performing simple descriptive estimates as the median, mean, range, and standard deviation before conducting exploration with more advanced multivariate statistics. The basic techniques are better suited to learning about properties such as the expected mean and data spread than are the multivariate techniques. A fundamental knowledge of the basic properties is important before applying more advanced methods.

5.4　Pattern Recognition and Clustering

Classification, clustering, and pattern recognition are different closely related terms that refer to statistical processes. They are used to specify samples in a set of categories. These categories can be prespecified (often referred to as supervised classification) or not prespecified (often referred to as unsupervised classification). In food science and nutrition classification, clustering, and pattern recognition have been used for, e.g., cultivar identification/classification based on geographical origin or variety, product identification/classification based on brand or plant, taxonomy and organism identification, and detection of adulteration.

Cluster analyses based on nearest-neighbor or hierarchical clusters are typical examples of unsupervised classification methods. The unsupervised approach can be used to determine if samples belong to classes not specified in advance. Mixture models constitute a more advanced set of methods often used in psychological research; they have also found application within the field of food science and nutrition, for example in the analysis of dietary patterns in epidemiological studies (Fahey et al. 2007). They are probabilistic models for representing the presence of subpopulations within an overall population.

The goal of so-called supervised methods is to assign new unknown objects (samples) to an existing class based on a classification rule. A training data set in which the classes of all samples are identified is used to calculate class boundaries and classification rules/models. The rule/model can then be applied to samples of unknown classes to predict their identity. Ideally, some samples should be reserved for a test data set and subject to the classification procedure to see if they are correctly classified. The degree of success in classifying samples is often evaluated by means of a misclassification matrix. This is a comparison of assigned (true) and predicted (from the classification rules developed) classes in a matrix. Correct results fall on a diagonal where the true class equals the predicted class.

Linear discriminant analysis is a classical technique for supervised classification and is also applied in food science. However, the technique has to a large extent been replaced by logistic regression, which does not assume that variables are normally distributed.

In chemometrics and its application to food science and nutrition, specialized methods such as soft independent modeling of class analogy (SIMCA) are sometimes used. SIMCA is mathematically related to PCA. It may be used on data with many highly correlated variables, such as, for example, spectrographic data, to perform a classification. The mathematical foundation of the method is, however, somewhat complex and outside the scope of this brief text. Interested readers may refer to the classical seminal paper by Wold (1976) or the textbook by Esbensen (2001) for a more detailed and mathematically technical description. These techniques are used, for example, within machine learning and chemometrics, but seems (yet) less applied on data from clinical studies. Methods based on PCA could make interpretation and the relationship with the original variables more complex. It could be argued that methods based on PCA should be used primarily when only an optimal classification is needed using highly correlated variables but without a detailed understanding of how each variable affects classification, as is often the case in medicine, psychology, or epidemiology.

5.5 Modeling and Optimization

Multivariate modeling and optimization are used in food production to assess the effects of raw materials and processing conditions on product quality. Another example of application areas of multivariate modeling is in determining the relationship between food products and sensory perceptions. Multivariate statistical techniques have been used in this capacity, for example, to assess the relationship between beverage constituents and haze and foam formation and in quantitative structure-activity relationship (QSAR) modeling of bioactive peptides, bitter taste, or functional properties such as foam or viscosity (Pripp et al. 2005; Siebert 2003)

Regression models are the statistical method of choice in modeling and optimization. The regression techniques typically used in food science include multiple linear regression (based on least-squares or maximum-likelihood estimation), PCR, or PLSR. Multiple linear regression is the most common regression method. It is linear in both the coefficients and predictors (measurements) and commonly described in statistical notation as

$$y = \beta_0 + \beta_1 \cdot x_1 + \beta_2 \cdot x_2 + ... + \beta_p \cdot x_p + \varepsilon$$

The β coefficients are calculated as the value that minimizes the residual sum of squares (or, equivalently, maximizes the log-likelihood function) and thus maximizes the correlation between a linear combination of predictors and the response. Multiple linear regression calculates an unbiased model but is sensitive to both outliers and highly correlated independent variables (multicollinearity). This regression method is used in many scientific areas.

The first step of PCR is to perform PCA as previously outlined. From a set of p variables a set q of principal components is estimated that accounts for a reasonably large part of the total variance:

$$PC_1 = \ell_{11}X_1 + \ell_{21}X_2 + ... + \ell_{p1}X_p$$
$$PC_2 = \ell_{12}X_1 + \ell_{22}X_2 + ... + \ell_{p2}X_p$$
$$\vdots$$
$$PC_q = \ell_{1q}X_1 + \ell_{2q}X_2 + ... + \ell_{p3}X_p$$

This produces scores and loadings as previously described. The scores are the values of each principal component for each sample, and the loadings are the subsequent coefficients multiplied by each initial variable for each principal component. The principal components are then treated as any other variable would be in a multiple linear regression analysis, and regression models are then constructed as

$$y = \beta_0 + \beta_1 \cdot PC_1 + \beta_2 \cdot PC_2 + ... + \beta_q \cdot PC_q + \varepsilon.$$

Principal components are calculated in their order of importance in terms of explaining the variance, and often the first one or two components will also best correlate with the dependent variable. However, this is not always the case. Since the principal components are orthogonal (no correlation), regression coefficients are unchanged with the inclusion of additional components in the model. PCR is well suited for prediction purposes with many correlated independent variables. If exploring the effect of each independent variable on the outcome is the goal, as is typical in many epidemiological or medical studies, then PCR may be of limited use. Thus, even though the regression equation from PCR is easily understood and applied to prediction, the relationship with the initial variables is much more obscure. This is the disadvantage of PCR and of the related PLSR method and, in many ways, all methods based on PCA. It is possible to assign an "interpretation" to each principal component, but the method is not designed to assess common underlying structures, and the interpretation of the principal components may not be straightforward and sometimes not even possible. PLSR is closely related to PCR. The conceptual difference is that PLSR calculates latent variables and regression coefficients at the same time. The latent variables are constructed to maximize their covariance with the dependent variables.

What is the problem with PLSR (and PCR) techniques, and why might additional caution be appropriate with their use in food science and nutrition? The first limitation is that they are linear models, but that applies to multiple linear regression as well. Linear models do tend to fit and explain many biological processes, and the transformation of variables may somewhat overcome this limitation. Another, more crucial, limitation has to do with the interpretation of latent variables and the relationship of the model with the initial measured variables. Interpretating and understanding the effect of the initial variables on a given outcome are often the main goal in the use of regression analysis in medicine and epidemiology. This may be why these methods are used less frequently in these fields. However, it may be argued that if interpretation – and not merely prediction – is the objective in food science and nutrition studies, then multiple regression methods could be more appropriate than PLSR or PCR. Perhaps PLSR and PCR should be limited to pure prediction models?

5.6 Limitations with Multivariate Statistical Analysis in Food Science

There is something very convincing with a simple statistical test! Multivariate statistical techniques, with all their scientific potential, multiple areas of application, and scientifically and intellectually stimulating properties, might not qualify as a simple statistical test; their complexity is often enhanced by extensive preprocessing of raw data in advance of statistical modeling (for a review on preprocessing see, e.g., Bro and Smilde 2003). This is the cost of using these methods. It is challenging to relate some of the findings to the original measurements. These methods should – in my opinion – not be the first line of data analysis of a new data set. The statistical-mathematical foundation of these techniques is extremely complicated and perhaps something that should be applied with caution, especially for those without training in the more basic techniques.

However, multivariate statistical techniques have several strengths when it comes to analyzing highly correlated data, prediction, data exploration, and their ability to analyze data sets with many variables compared to samples – as is increasingly the case in many fields of research. They could therefore be expected to find increased application within clinical and medical research as well.

References

Bro R, Smilde AK (2003) Centering and scaling in component analysis. J Chemometr 17:16–33. doi:10.1002/cem.773

Esbensen KH (2001) Multivariate data analysis – in practice. An introduction to multivariate data analysis and experimental design, 5th edn. CAMO ASA, Oslo

Fabrigar LR, Wegener DT, MacCallum RC, Strahan EJ (1999) Evaluating the use of exploratory factor analysis in psychological research. Psychol Methods 4:272–299. doi:10.1037/1082-989X.4.3.272

Fahey MT, Thane CW, Bramwell GD, Coward WA (2007) Conditional gaussian mixture modeling for dietary patterns. J R Stat Soc Ser A-G 170:149–166. doi:10.1111/j.1467-985X.2006.00452.x

Johnson RA, Wichern DW (2007) Applied multivariate statistical analysis, 6th edn. Pearson Prentice Hall, Upper Saddle River

Kahn JH (2006) Factor analysis in counseling psychology research, training and practice: principles, advances, and applications. Couns Psychol 34:684–718. doi:10.1177/0011000006286347

Karoui R, Baerdemaeker JD (2007) A review of the analytical methods coupled with chemometric tools for the determination of the quality and identity of dairy products. Food Chem 102:621–640. doi:10.1016/j.foodchem.2006.05.042

Kozak M, Scaman CH (2008) Unsupervised classification methods in food sciences: discussion and outlook. J Sci Food Agric 88:1115–1127. doi:10.1002/jsfa.3215

Pripp AH, Isaksson T, Stepaniak L, Sørhaug T, Ardö Y (2005) Quantitative structure activity relationship modelling of peptides and proteins as a tool in food science. Trends Food Sci Technol 16:484–494. doi:10.1016/j.tifs.2005.07.003

Siebert KJ (2003) Modeling protein functional properties from amino acid composition. J Agric Food Chem 51:7792–7797. doi:10.1021/jf0342775

Suhr D (2009) Principal component analysis vs. exploratory factor analysis. SUGI 30 proceedings. http://www2.sas.com/proceedings/sugi30/203-30.pdf. Accessed 5 Jun 2012

Tzouros NE, Arvanitoyannis IS (2001) Agricultural produces: synopsis of employed quality control methods for the authentication of foods and application of chemometrics for the classification of foods according to their variety of geographical origin. Crit Rev Food Sci Nutr 41:287–319. doi:10.1080/20014091091823

Widaman KF (1993) Common factor-analysis versus principal component analysis – differential bias in representing model parameters. Multivar Behav Res 28:263–311. doi:10.1207/s15327906mbr2803_1

Wold S (1976) Pattern-recognition by means of disjoint principal components models. Pattern Recognit 8:127–139. doi:10.1016/0031-3203(76)90014-5

Statistics in Food Science and Nutrition

Are Hugo Pripp

A.H. Pripp, *Statistics in Food Science and Nutrition*, SpringerBriefs in Food,
Health, and Nutrition, DOI 10.1007/978-1-4614-5010-8,
© Springer Science+Business Media New York 2013

DOI 10.1007/978-1-4614-5010-8_6

The copyright holder of the Springer Brief *Statistics in Food Science and Nutrition* is incorrectly given as Springer instead of the author, Are Hugo Pripp. Consequently, the copyright holder should appear as: © Are Hugo Pripp 2013.

The online version of the original book can be found at
http://dx.doi.org/10.1007/978-1-4614-5010-8

Index

A.H. Pripp, *Statistics in Food Science and Nutrition*, SpringerBriefs in Food,
Health, and Nutrition, DOI 10.1007/978-1-4614-5010-8,
© Springer Science+Business Media New York 2013